Non-Heart-Beating Organ Transplantation

Medical and Ethical Issues in Procurement

Division of Health Care Services

INSTITUTE OF MEDICINE

Roger Herdman, *Study Director,* and
John T. Potts, *Principal Investigator*

NATIONAL ACADEMY PRESS
Washington, D.C. 1997

NATIONAL ACADEMY PRESS • 2101 Constitution Avenue, N.W. • Washington, DC 20418

NOTICE: The project that is the subject of this report was approved by the Governing Board of the National Research Council, whose members are drawn from the councils of the National Academy of Sciences, the National Academy of Engineering, and the Institute of Medicine.

This report has been reviewed by a group other than the authors according to procedures approved by a Report Review Committee consisting of members of the National Academy of Sciences, the National Academy of Engineering, and the Institute of Medicine.

The Institute of Medicine was chartered in 1970 by the National Academy of Sciences to enlist distinguished members of the appropriate professions in the examination of policy matters pertaining to the health of the public. In this, the Institute acts under the Academy's 1863 congressional charter responsibility to be an adviser to the federal government and its own initiative in identifying issues of medical care, research, and education. Dr. Kenneth I. Shine is president of the Institute of Medicine.

Support for this project was provided by the U.S. Department of Health and Human Services (Contract No. 240-97-0012). The opinions expressed in this report are those of the authors and do not necessarily reflect the views of the sponsor.

International Standard Book No. 0-309-06424-4

Additional copies of *Non-Heart-Beating Organ Transplantation: Medical and Ethical Issues in Procurement* are available for sale from the National Academy Press, 2101 Constitution Avenue, N.W., Box 285, Washington, DC 20055. Call (800) 624-6242 or (202) 334-3313 (in the Washington metropolitan area) or visit the NAP's on-line bookstore at **www.nap.edu**.

For more information about the Institute of Medicine, visit the IOM home page at **www2.nas.edu/iom**.

Copyright 1997 by the National Academy of Sciences. All rights reserved.

Printed in the United States of America.

The serpent has been a symbol of long life, healing, and knowledge among almost all cultures and religions since the beginning of recorded history. The serpent adopted as a logotype by the Institute of Medicine is a relief carving from ancient Greece, now held by the Staatliche Museen in Berlin.

PRINCIPAL INVESTIGATOR

JOHN T. POTTS, Jr., M.D., Distinguished Jackson Professor of Clinical Medicine and Director of Research, Massachusetts General Hospital, Boston

Staff

ROGER HERDMAN, M.D., Study Director
KATHLEEN NOLAN, Research Assistant
HEATHER CALLAHAN, Program Assistant
INGRID BURGER, Research Assistant

Preface

In the spring of 1997, the Department of Health and Human Services (DHHS) contacted the Institute of Medicine (IOM) to express concern about the national state of organ donation and the supply of solid organs for transplantation to patients with terminal organ failures. Questions had been raised recently about the management of cadaver donors who died a cardiopulmonary death, called non-heart-beating donors (NHBDs). These questions focused on whether interventions undertaken in these donors to enhance the supply and quality of solid organs for transplantation were in the best interests of the donor patient or were, in fact, hastening death. Anticoagulants and vasodilators were singled out in particular for examination, but a subsequent letter from DHHS's general counsel (see Appendix A) framed the issue in more general terms: "Given a potential donor in an end-of-life situation, what are the alternative medical approaches that can be used to maximize the availability of organs from that donor without violating prevailing ethical norms regarding the rights and welfare of donors: The Institute will consider the alternative approaches, including the use of anti-coagulants or vasodilators, from the scientific as well as the ethical point of view." Proper answers to these questions are necessary to maintain a successful national organ procurement and transplantation program that enjoys the confidence of, and attracts organ donation from, the American public.

This report defines the various kinds of organ donors, including the four categories of NHBDs, and discusses the large and growing gap between supply and demand for donors and solid organs. The long, evolving history of NHBDs in transplantation is reviewed, and the data on current and potential supply, clinical results, and cost-effectiveness of these donors are presented. Also reported are the results of a survey of the NHBD protocols and activities of the 63 U.S. organ procurement organizations active in the late spring of 1997. The issues that flow from the information collected on this subject matter and that are relevant to the DHHS charge are identified. The data and issues are analyzed for the purposes of framing conclusions and recommendations that will illuminate the questions of alternative approaches and ethical and scientific norms mentioned in the department's letter.

This report represents a new kind of effort by the IOM, that is, a report not by a committee but using a principal investigator (PI) model. The IOM asked John T. Potts, Jr., M.D., Distinguished Jackson Professor of Clinical Medicine and director of research, Massachusetts General Hospital, Boston, to serve as the principal investigator. "The National Academy of Sciences (NAS), the National Academy of Engineering (NAE), and the Institute of Medicine jointly administer the work of the National Research Council (NRC) in rendering independent advice to the federal government on scientific and technical matters. The current portfolio of activities in the Academy Complex reflects a variety of approaches in fulfilling this mission, including the use of principal investigators. PIs are appointed by the NRC chair. The plan for the conduct of an IOM study using PIs will generally include opportunities for soliciting the individual views of other scientific and technical experts and for public input via written comments and/or public hearings. The PIs are tasked with preparing a draft NRC or IOM report that represents the state of scientific and technical knowledge concerning the issues under investigation. The draft IOM report will be examined in accordance with the usual rigorous review procedures of the Academy and appropriately revised before being approved for release to the sponsor and the public."*

A number of senior special experts were asked to provide their professional expertise and experience to inform and support this work. The IOM deeply appreciates the exemplary performance of all of these individuals. Their contributions to and support of this report enhance its value. They are recognized and their efforts described at the beginning of this report. It is important that these individuals are neither transplant personnel, nor members of, or directly involved with, transplant or organ procurement programs. They are independent experts in various fields of medicine, ethics, and the law and are generally knowledgeable about, but "at arm's length from," transplantation.

Leading figures in the transplant community, federal government, and donor family and recipient groups, without exception, responded to the IOM's need for information from those with front-line, detailed experience and expertise in matters of solid organ procurement and transplantation. These individuals are noted and their contributions described in Appendix B. The opportunity given to the principal investigator, senior special experts, and IOM staff thereby was essential in providing a time to question and learn about real-world activi-

---

*Principal Investigator Model (Updated 10/21/97). Section 3: Projects at the National Academy Complex Involving Principal Investigators (slightly edited).

ties in transplantation. The IOM greatly appreciates the willingness of these individuals to assist this work.

Others who were particularly helpful and made important contributions to this study include the leadership of the United Network for Organ Sharing (UNOS): Walter Graham, Mary Ellison, O. Patrick Daily, and Doug Heiney and its immediate past president, James Burdick. UNOS provided special summaries of national data not otherwise available. The IOM appreciates the assistance of Stephen Rose, Dan Rotrosen, and Nancy Blustein of the National Institute of Allergy and Infectious Disease and of Judith Braslow, Remy Aronoff, and Gwen Mayes of the Division of Transplantation, Health Resources and Services Administration. Jimmy Light and Anne Kowalski also provided important help, as did Stuart Youngner, Roger Evans, Carol Beasley, Richard Rettig, Tim Henderson, Lana Price, Sandy Zachary, Henry Desmarais, Louise Jacobbi, John Fung, Mel Worth, and Robert Epstein. The IOM received outstanding cooperation from the 63 U.S. organ procurement organizations. The information supplied by them and reported here in the survey in chapter 5 provided a picture of the state of affairs in NHBD organ procurement across the entire country that was vital to consideration of the questions the IOM was asked to address.

The financial support of this work by the Department of Health and Human Services, in particular the strong interest and support of the Division of Transplantation, is gratefully acknowledged. Additional support was provided from internal funds of the Institute of Medicine. Institute staff who worked on this report were Roger Herdman, Kathleen Nolan, Heather Callahan, and Ingrid Burger.

ACKNOWLEDGMENTS

Senior Special Experts

The following Senior Special Experts attended and analyzed presentations from transplant and organ procurement experts on July 30, 1997. Based on this information, data provided by IOM staff, and their own experience and expertise in the fields of anesthesiology, bioethics, cardiology, critical care, law, medicine, neurology, nursing, physiology, and surgery, they provided advice to the principal investigator and IOM staff, discussed issues and recommendations, and reviewed early drafts of the report.

FRANCOIS M. ABBOUD, M.D., Professor of Medicine and Physiology and of Biophysics; Chairman of Medicine; Edith King Pearson Professor of Cardiovascular Research; and Director, Cardiovascular Research Center, University of Iowa College of Medicine

TOM L. BEAUCHAMP, Ph.D., Professor of Bioethics, Kennedy Institute of Ethics, Georgetown University

ROBERT M. BERNE, M.D., Professor of Physiology, Emeritus, University of Virginia Health Sciences Center

BARBARA J. DALY, Ph.D., R.N., Associate Professor, Case Western Reserve University School of Nursing

ROBERT J. JOYNT, M.D., Ph.D., Distinguished University Professor and Professor of Neurology, University of Rochester

JOHN P. KAMPINE, M.D., Ph.D., Professor and Chairman, Department of Anesthesiology, Medical College of Wisconsin

LASALLE D. LEFFALL, Jr., M.D., Charles R. Drew Professor of Surgery, Department of Surgery, Howard University College of Medicine

JOHN A. ROBERTSON, J.D., Thomas Watt Gregory Professor of Law, University of Texas at Austin School of Law

Contents

EXECUTIVE SUMMARY 1

1 **INTRODUCTION** 7

2 **TRANSPLANTATION SUPPLY AND DEMAND** 10
   Supply, 10
   Demand, 11
   Improving Supply, 14

3 **BACKGROUND** 20
   The Historical Non-Heart-Beating Donor, 20
   Neurologic Criteria for Death, 21

4 **THE MODERN NON-HEART-BEATING DONOR** 23
   The Controlled NHBD, 23
   The Uncontrolled NHBD, 25
   Current Status of the NHBD in Transplantation, 26

5 **SURVEY OF ORGAN PROCUREMENT ORGANIZATION AND TRANSPLANT PROGRAM POLICIES** 33
   Interest in OPO NHBD Protocols, 34
   Protocol Statistics, 34
   Identification of Potential Donors, 35
   Approach to Family for Consent, 37
   OPO and Procurement Team Intervention Before Death, 38
   Medication, 39
   Withdrawal of Life Support and Declaration of Death, 40

Withdrawal of Life Support and Declaration of Death, 40
Uncontrolled NHBDs, 42
Conclusion, 43

6 ANALYSIS, FINDINGS, AND RECOMMENDATIONS 45
General Principles, 45
Policies and Oversight, 47
Medical Interventions and Ethics, 50
Conflicts of Interest, 55
Determination of Death, 57
Families, 61

REFERENCES 65

APPENDIXES
A Letter to the Institute of Medicine from the Department of Health and Human Services, 73
B Agenda and Summary of Workshop on Medical and Ethical Issues in Maintaining the Viability of Organs for Transplantation, 75
C U.S. Organ Procurement Organizations and Letter of Request for Non-Heart-Beating Donor Protocols, 89

Executive Summary

This report examines medical and ethical issues in recovering organs from non-heart-beating donors (NHBDs) who do not meet the standard of brain death. These are patients who are either severely ill on life support, and life support can be withdrawn with proper consent, or they have suffered unexpected cardiac arrest, whether previously ill or not, and cannot be resuscitated. These patients are called, respectively, controlled or uncontrolled NHBDs—controlled because death and organ removal can be predictably controlled and planned following withdrawal of life support; uncontrolled because the occurrence of cardiac arrest is unplanned and the timing and some other aspects of organ removal are not controlled; and non-heart-beating because death is determined by cessation of heart and respiratory function, not whole brain function.

This report makes recommendations to implement the following general conclusion: the recovery of organs from NHBDs is an important, medically effective, and ethically acceptable approach to reducing the gap that exists now and will exist in the future between the demand for and the available supply of organs for transplantation. Discussions and media reports about recovery of organs from NHBDs arising from the Pittsburgh protocol and the Cleveland Clinic proposal have generated questions about whether the use of organs from NHBDs raises unique or insurmountable ethical problems. The problems raised require attention, but they are, in fact, not significantly different from those that arise in cadaveric transplantation generally. The design and implementation of standards and procedural guidelines for organ recovery from NHBDs based on the principles that support the retrieval of organs from brain-dead donors, would address these problems and allow the development of non-heart-beating organ donation as an important source of organs for transplantation. Such an enhancement of organ donation would be of significant societal value.

Solid organ transplantation activities in the United States include health care financing, program assistance, oversight, and research support from the Department of Health and Human Services (DHHS). National data collection, analysis, and reporting and allocation of organs from the United Network for Organ Sharing; donor procurement by more than 60 organ procurement organizations working with about 1,300 donor hospitals; and health care delivery in about 275 transplant centers—all of which make up the national Organ Procurement and Transplantation Network—are also part of transplantation services. In addition, there are organizations of physicians and other procurement and transplant personnel, recipients, and donor families among other groups that support and advocate transplantation. Much of this activity is pursuant to federal, state, or local law and regulation.

This effort exists because of, and cannot succeed without, members of the public, who donate organs for transplantation. During life, they volunteer as living donors or execute donor cards or other advance directives to provide organs at death, or in the absence of directives, at death their families consent to the removal of organs for transplantation. Unfortunately, this national effort is inadequate in the sense that donor numbers are growing only slowly at the same time that demand for organs increasingly exceeds the supply. This is happening as research has led to a better understanding of transplantation biology and transplantation technology and results have been consistently improving. The current situation demands enhanced organ recovery from traditional donors, the exploration of new approaches to organ donation and recovery, and the implementation of national donor procurement and care standards that adhere strictly to ethical and scientific norms and will reinforce public confidence in the donor process.

This study is the Institute of Medicine's response to a request from the DHHS. That request, in essence, posed the general question, how can the United States have a good organ donor and transplantation program? The actual request letter (see Appendix A) was focused more specifically and circumscribed the question to, what are the alternative medical approaches that can be used to increase the availability of organs and at the same time ensure the ethically and medically sound treatment of donor patients before and after death? The IOM was also asked to review some specific interventions that are undertaken in donors to preserve organs for transplantation, such as the administration of anticoagulants and vasodilators. Furthermore, the DHHS request focused the study on very severely ill or injured, but not brain dead, patients with informed consent for withdrawal of life support (primarily mechanical ventilation) or patients who suffer cardiac arrest and cannot be resuscitated, called, as noted earlier, respectively, controlled and uncontrolled NHBDs.

The premises that organ transplantation is a valuable treatment that should be supported and extended to all suitable patients with organ failure and that organs from NHBDs are an underutilized, although potentially very significant, source of organs for transplantation that deserves careful exploration were starting points for this report. The data on total organ supply from all kinds of donors, the national demand for organs, the disparity between supply and demand, and the avenues that might be taken to improve supply from existing kinds of donors are explored. Analysis of the evidence suggests that supply could and should be enhanced but that, without scientific breakthroughs, demand probably always will exceed the organs available from human sources.

The four different categories of NHBDs (one controlled and three uncontrolled) are described in this report, and the most recent data on U.S. transplantation with these donors along with the results, which are comparable to results of transplants involving organs recovered from brain-dead patients, are reported. The background material includes a short history of organ transplantation in the United States, and reviews development of the definition and criteria for brain death and of the state laws for defining death as cessation of function of either the whole brain or the circulatory and respiratory systems. The point is made that there is an unmet need for organs, as well as scientific and clinical justification and historical precedent that support an exploration of the alternatives to increase organ availability including recovery of organs from NHBDs.

The analysis of the potential role of these donors in transplantation includes a survey of all 63 current organ procurement organizations and the NHBD protocols that have been approved or are under development in 34 of them. This analysis describes variations and contradictions among protocols and—within the context of a set of identified principles—provides a framework for organizing the issues and recommendations involved. The principles identified indicate the ways in which viable organs can best be recovered from NHBDs in a manner that is consistent with appropriate medical and ethical standards. The main principles, or general approaches, which are relevant to all cadaveric donors including NHBDs, are summarized in Box 1. The five headings used to organize the issues are (1) policies and oversight, (2) medical interventions and ethics, (3) conflicts of interest, (4) determination of death, and (5) families.

Box 1
Principles

1. The societal value of enhancing organ donation.
2. Organ donors must be dead at organ removal.
3. Absolute prohibition of active euthanasia.
4. Complete openness about policies and protocols.
5. Commitment to informed consent.
6. Respect for donor and family wishes.

> **Box 2**
> **Recommendations for National Policy**
>
> 1. Written, locally approved NHBD protocols.
> 2. Public openness of NHBD protocols.
> 3. Case by case decisions on anticoagulants and vasodilators.
> 4. Family consent for premortem cannulation.
> 5. Conflict of interest safeguards—separate times and personnel for important decisions.
> 6. Determination of death in controlled NHBDs by cessation of cardiopulmonary function for at least 5 minutes by electrocardiographic and arterial pressure monitoring.
> 7. Family options (e.g., attendance at life support withdrawal) and financial protection.

Local policies and protocols may appropriately reflect local differences in custom and practice. There should, however, be some national uniformity. Outright contradictions—for example, a blanket prohibition of anticoagulants and vasodilators as hastening death in one case and their routine administration to living donors before withdrawal of life support in other cases, citing the inadequacy of pulse palpation for determining death in one case and relying on it in another, or using different definitions of death—are not likely to engender public confidence in the management of NHBDs. Although the consequences of these inconsistencies may be more perceived than real, this report recommends that they be resolved. The recommendations that are important for national policy are summarized in Box 2 and this section of the report. They are described in greater detail in the Analysis section of this report. First of all, **protocols should be open, public documents**, and given the ethical and medical complexity of NHBDs, **organ procurement should be carried out only after advance thought and planning that has been reduced to a written protocol developed with public input (including the views of patient and donor families) and approved by appropriate local oversight bodies.**

The medical-ethical issues specific to the DHHS request concerned administration of the anticoagulant heparin and the vasodilator phentolamine (Regitine™). The NHBD protocols reviewed are divided evenly between allowing the use at some stage in the donation process of one or both of these agents and expressly prohibiting or not mentioning them. In most cases, careful administration is appropriate. Nevertheless, because under certain circumstances in certain patients, there is a concern that these agents might be harmful, this report recommends **case-by-case decisions on the use of anticoagulants and vasodilators,** and consideration of additional safeguards such as involvement of the patient's attending physician in prescribing decisions. Major vascular cannulation for organ perfusion with cooling and preserving solutions is discussed. **Premortem cannulation of controlled NHBDs is acceptable, but requires** informed family consent. The pros and cons of postmortem cannulation in potential donors without consent are presented. This issue remains open. In the absence of a clear ethical resolution, the best policy may be to require consent.

This report discusses and reinforces the **safeguards against conflicts of interest.** These include **separating decisions about and management of care with respect to life support withdrawal and donation, determination of death and organ removal by appropriate timing and by keeping the responsibilities of attending patient care physicians and other personnel separate from those of transplant or procurement physicians and personnel.** Also discussed are the difficulties of eliminating "institutional" biases toward donation and transplantation in settings such as transplant hospitals where there are institutional advantages to increasing donor and transplant numbers.

As noted earlier, the definitions of death and standards for determining death differ in protocols across the country. Defining death is a matter for state law and may vary. However, defining and determining death are much more critical in organ donors than in other patients. In heart-beating, brain-dead donors there is a need for clear understanding and implementation of the criteria for brain death to ensure that the donor patient is dead. Concerns of organ viability are relieved by continued circulation. In NHBDs there is a requirement to ensure that the donor patient is dead so as to avoid even the perception of organ removal from a living person, but at the same time, to bring removal as close as possible to the cessation of circulatory and respiratory function in order to ensure organs in the most viable condition. Existing NHBD protocols either are unclear or specify organ removal from immediately to 5 minutes after heart stoppage. In view of the critical nature of this decision, **this report recommends that not less than a 5-minute interval, determined accurately by electronic and arterial pulse pressure monitoring, be required to determine donor death in controlled NHBDs. No recommendations are made for uncontrolled NHBDs, and for the time being, details of how to define and determine death in these donors are left to the judgment of local medical experts.**

This report strongly encourages discretion and sensitivity with respect to the circumstances, views, and beliefs of families (language of U.S. Code 42: 1320b-8(a)(1)(A)). **Families need to be fully informed, given privacy and time to adjust, and provided with the option of attending the withdrawal of life support and the death of their loved ones.** Appropriate follow-up after donation and the Bill of Rights for Donor Families are discussed and supported. Some NHBD protocols contain explicit guarantees that donors will not incur costs. **Donors and their families should not suffer financial penalties by altruistically contributing to the national donation effort.**

Not all issues were addressed in this study that could have been, and as noted, some that were raised have been left for future discussion. Changes in the nationwide transplant effort described and recommended here (and summarized in Box 2) should be made. The process could involve participation by the transplant community, donor families, recipients, and the public in consultative roles. An open process to identify and address problems is important because public perceptions of deficiencies in the care of NHBDs can damage ongoing organ recovery efforts and because organs donated by families of NHBDs can provide a potentially important contribution to efforts to bring organ supply closer to demand.

1

Introduction

This report is about transplanting solid organs—primarily kidneys but also livers and to a lesser extent hearts, pancreases, and lungs—from cadavers to recipients in whom one or more of these organs have failed. The focus is on organs recovered from cadavers under specific circumstances. These cadavers are called non-heart-beating donors (NHBDs)* to distinguish them from the more usual brain-dead† (but heart-beating) and living, healthy donors. The report, most importantly, is concerned with identifying and addressing the issues raised in consideration of the NHBD as part of the effort to achieve the valuable goal of an organ supply that is closer to demand and yet to remain within the ethical boundaries that ensure the rights and welfare of donor patients.

The ethical and legal requirements for donor patient care and the imperatives of the organ conservation, recovery, and transplant process seem to render actions on behalf of donors as patients and as donors, and on behalf of organs that are in condition to give recipients the best possible chance for new hope and life, difficult or even impossible to reconcile. The issues raised by these actions

---

*Although "donor" is standard usage, most NHBDs are not donors as the word is usually understood outside of this context, because they themselves did not consent. Instead, their responsible family members or a legal surrogate gave permission for organ donation. Nevertheless, the words "donor" or "donation" are generally understood in this context, and possible replacements like recovery, removal, retrieval, and procurement are not synonyms, do not capture the sense of altruism implicit in "donation," and in practice are unwieldy to use uniformly. Thus the words "donor" and "donation" are used in this report with the knowledge that they recognize the gift but inaccurately attribute it.

†"Brain-dead" is legally identical to "dead." The unnecessary and confusing modifier serves the practical purpose of specifying which legal determination of the primary cause of death, whole brain or cardiopulmonary, is meant.

and the responses they have engendered are identified and addressed later in this report on the medical and ethical issues in procuring organs for transplantation. They are also the ones that have occupied the biomedical and ethics communities in clinical and research efforts to solve them. These issues are particularly salient in the NHBD because interventions in the heart-beating donor occur in a brain-dead cadaver, and the living donor involves an autonomous, consenting person for whom every effort in his or her care is addressed toward a healthy, medically uncompromised survival.

There is a relentlessly increasing need for organs for patients with life-threatening organ failures that requires the recruitment of donors and timely intervention to obtain the donated organs in the best possible transplantable condition. Delay because of insufficient organ supply proves fatal to one-third of waiting heart and liver recipients. The total number of waiting list deaths now exceeds 4,000 each year, and for all those waiting, morbidity, pain, depression, and economic costs are a constant part of their lives (Perkins, 1987; UNOS, 1996; Youngner and Arnold, 1993).

At the same time, persons who have been or may be designated as donors have, during a final illness, rights to health care that meets appropriate, prevailing medical and ethical standards (Sadler et al., 1968). This care must promote the individual's welfare and provide the best chance for recovery, no matter how small, or for a death with as much comfort and dignity as possible. Any exceptions to the principle that decisions about, and the administration of, health care should be separate from, and uninfluenced by, any considerations of transplantation must be explicit, ethical, and subject to informed consent. Donor patients must not be killed or their death hastened by the taking of organs (the "dead donor rule," which operationally has meant that donors must be dead before donation). Furthermore, their welfare and care must not be compromised by preparation for organ retrieval, and the sensitivity and grief of family and friends must be respected. These considerations and principles apply to all kinds of cadaver donors, and they must be preserved in the face of the interventions desirable to obtain organs in the best transplantable condition. The best organs are those that are perfused by warm, oxygenated blood up to the very moment of their removal from the donor's body. These conditions are met only in heart-beating—that is, living and brain-dead—donors. Attempts to approach or simulate these ideal conditions for recovery of organs from NHBDs, therefore, pose challenges that are complex and in certain respects different from those of other donors.

The preferred NHBD in the United States is the "controlled" NHBD. Those caring for and carrying out transplantation from controlled NHBDs must manage patients with severe injury or disease, usually involving the brain, who do not meet the legal test for death by neurologic criteria and whose cardiopulmonary function has been resuscitated or is being supported through medical technology. Physicians must maintain as normal as possible blood and oxygen supply to organs, provide organ-conserving interventions as necessary, discontinue breathing and circulatory support when a proper decision and proper consent to do so has been obtained to allow the irreversible cessation of cardiac and pulmonary function so as to meet the legal standard of death, and then begin preserving and removing organs as soon as possible before they deteriorate. This tightly scheduled management of the donor patient and the transplantable organs must, as noted, satisfy a number of important ethical principles, including the dead donor rule, respect for family wishes, prohibition against euthanasia, and informed consent.

To some extent in this country, and more often in Europe, transplantation involves a category of NHBDs who are not controlled by technological support of respiration and heart function. These individuals (uncontrolled NHBDs) have suffered cardiopulmonary arrest as a result of severe illness or injury just before admission or during their hospital stay. This "uncontrolled" event dictates great speed in retrieving organs, early organ preservation interventions, or sequences of resuscitation efforts that start and stop depending on the status of the donor and the transplantable organs. This process must meet ethical principles similar to those for controlled NHBDs. Because the medical and ethical issues and the problems of all NHBDs, controlled or uncontrolled, are similar in so many essential ways, this report should and does examine all categories of NHBD.

2

Transplantation Supply and Demand

SUPPLY

Transplantation data from the United Network for Organ Sharing (UNOS) counts 8,940 total donors for the most recent year reported (1996), of which 5,416 were cadaver donors and 3,524 were living donors. Over the last 9 years (1988 to 1996), the total number of donors (5,910 to 8,940, up 51%), cadaver donors (4,084 to 5,416, up 33%) and living donors (1,827 to 3,524, up 93%) has been increasing slowly (UNOS-Organ Procurement and Transplantation Network (OPTN)/Scientific Registry data as of July 5, 1997). This increase is not due to NHBDs. Their numbers at present are very small and do not influence these figures (see UNOS data later in this chapter).

Increased supply has come about in three principal ways: (1) There are more living donors, and among these spouses and friends who are emotionally as opposed to genetically related donors increased from 3.9% to 12.5% of all living donors from 1988 to 1996. (2) Criteria for accepting cadaver donors have begun to be liberalized and expanded to include, importantly, increasing age (up to 80 years) in some programs, but also donors with diabetes, hypertension, some infections, high-risk social history but negative HIV test, some hemodynamic instability, some chemical imbalances, increased organ preservation time by perfusion or storage using cold solutions, or increased time after death in the body. These expanded criteria are said to have the potential to add 25 to 39% to the cadaver donor supply (Briceno et al., 1997; Jacobbi et al., 1997). In 1996, donors over age 50 comprised 26.5% of all U.S. cadaver donors, double the 1990 percentage (Braslow, 1997). (3) Lastly, there is more efficient use of each donor; that is, more solid organs are procured (and transplanted) per donor. The donor–transplant ratio for living donors, from whom only those organs that are paired or removable in part can be taken, is always about 1. The ratio for cadaver donors, from whom all solid organs can be taken, rose, in terms of not only organs procured per donor (21%, from 2.98 to 3.60) but as organs actually transplanted per donor (18%, from 2.73 to 3.21 from 1988 to 1996)* (OPTN/Scientific Registry data as of April 15, 1997). Unfortunately, no improvement in the organ-per-donor figures has occurred since 1993, and the organ-per-donor yield for NHBDs is, and likely will remain, lower as that category is expanded (2.5 organs-per-donor, and 1.78 transplants-per-donor, aggregate from 1993 to 1996) (M. Ellison, personal communication, June 27, 1997).

These comparative numbers of transplants or recipients per donor should be part of an assessment of supply and demand. Also the success of transplantation—the survival of the transplanted organ and the recipient patient—depends heavily on the condition of the donor organ (Cosio et al., 1997; Light et al., 1996; Jacobbi et al., 1997). The expansion of criteria for acceptance of organs from donors of greater age and in less satisfactory medical conditions and the increased use of NHBDs exact a price in increased procurement costs of 23% more per donor and thus even more per organ (L. Jacobbi, personal communication, July 17, 1997); increased cost of transplantation; and lower graft (i.e., the transplanted organ) and recipient survival (Alexander et al., 1994; Briceno et al., 1997; Casavilla et al., 1996; Jacobbi et al., 1997; Light et al., 1996; Whiting et al., 1997). This must be weighed against the morbidity, death, and economic and other costs in patients on the waiting list (Hauptman and O'Connor, 1997; Perkins, 1987; Light et al., 1996).

Regardless of donor type, overall patient and graft survival rates have continued to improve over time. One-year graft survivals now range from 74% to 92% depending on the organ, although in subsequent years survivals gradually decrease particularly in expanded donor and NHBD transplants. The best results are with kidneys, which comprised 51% of all cadaver transplants and 98% of all living donor transplants in 1996 (OPTN/Scientific Registry data as of July 5, 1997). Coincident with improvements in the technology available and these better results, the pool of potential recipients has been expanding steadily (Anaise and Rapaport, 1993). These trends are likely to continue.

DEMAND

Changes in supply should be compared with changes in demand. The transplantation waiting list contained 50,047 people waiting on the last day of 1996, 14% more than the previous year and 212% more than at the end of 1988

---

*The difference between organs procured and organs transplanted (the discard rate) is the loss caused primarily by various medical and viability problems in removed organs that makes them unsuitable for transplantation. Greater use of donors accepted under expanded criteria and NHBDs is causing a rising discard rate.

(16,026). During that 9-year interval, 23,214 people died while on the waiting list—4,083 people in 1996 alone. Most median waits (the number of days elapsing until 50% of those waiting receive a transplant) have been increasing; the most recent are as follows: for kidneys (1994), 842 days; for livers (1995), 254 days; and for hearts (1995), 213 days (UNOS, 1996). These data have recently been superseded by not yet published waits stratified by recipient status: for example, median waits are 609 days, 1,046 days, and "too long to have a median at present" in the least, moderately, and most severely sensitized kidney recipients, respectively. They range from 5 days in the sickest liver recipients to 311 days for those liver candidates in the best condition and, similarly, from 40 to 390 days for the sickest to the healthiest heart recipients. These unpublished data emphasize that waiting times depend largely on candidate medical conditions. They also reflect, for heart and liver, the positive effects of preferences accorded to the most severely ill recipients (M. Ellison, personal communication, July 5, 1997).

In 1996, 33,866 patients were added to the waiting list, and 20,319 organ transplants were performed and removed that number of patients from the waiting list. Death removed 4,083 patients from the list, as noted earlier. An additional 1,019 patients were removed from the list due to advanced disease, and 1,941 patients left the list because of improved status, refusal of transplantation, and other unspecified reasons (OPTN/Scientific Registry data as of July 29, 1997). At a steady state, therefore, it would appear that conforming demand—as measured by the addition of new patients to the list, deaths, and removals from the list due to advanced disease—with supply—as measured by number of transplants performed—would require an increase in organs of around 18,000 (about 90%) and, depending on the kind of donor, because of varying numbers of organs recovered per donor, about the same percentage increase in donors. Without the need to overcome this large backlog, such an equilibrium—even if supply could in some way be increased by the requisite amount—is unlikely for several reasons.

Many observers believe that there are potential recipients who could benefit from transplantation, but because the supply situation is so daunting, through a kind of informal rationing they are not added to the waiting list and therefore are not included on the demand side (Caplan, 1986). Furthermore, 1991 demand estimates based on disease incidence suggested a greater potential need, in the neighborhood of twice the then-current new patient additions to the waiting list (Evans et al., 1992). If estimates are accurate that 30%–40% of patients on hemodialysis are suitable transplant candidates, there should be 60,048 to 80,064 of the 200,160 End Stage Renal Disease Program 1995 roster on the waiting list, but the actual number awaiting kidney transplant on December 31, 1995 was only 31,195 (Anaise and Rapaport, 1993; Health Care Financing Administration, 1997). A recent estimate of suitable heart recipients of 14,000 per year greatly exceeds the 1996 heart transplant (2,368) and waiting list

(3,648) totals (Federle, 1995; OPTN/Scientific Registry data as of July 29, 1997), and the most recent estimate by Roger Evans of unmet need in 1996 was 121,200 (personal communication, August 14, 1997). As noted elsewhere, changes in many parameters—medical technology, disease patterns, expanded indications for transplantation, transplant success rates, funding for health care, the general supply of, and access to transplant services, and the organization of the general health care system and the organ procurement system—will also influence any equilibrium. Better results make transplantation more sought after, more transplant centers make it more easily accessible, and all of these factors influence physicians' perceptions of the indications for referral for this treatment.

Because the available data document the fact that demand is increasing significantly faster than supply and has been for some time (donor increase, 1988–1996, 51%; waiting list increase, 1988–1996, 212%), an equilibrium on the waiting list achieved through increased waiting times and higher death rates, accompanied by increased morbidity and economic and other costs, seems the inevitable, ultimate result of current trends. These adverse effects will occur not only among those on the list, but are likely too among those who receive transplants because they will have waited much longer, will have advanced disability and disease, and will be less medically suitable transplant candidates. Three-year graft survivals for liver and heart patients who are not hospitalized versus those needing life support are 24% and 9% higher, respectively, and transplant procedure charges are respectively 84% and 68% higher for those needing life support (R. Evans, personal communication, August 14, 1997).

Demand could be limited by an explicit decision to ration services by narrowing the indications for transplantation, a decision that would be extremely difficult and controversial in its details. The implicit rationing, noted above, could continue in an informally and tacitly expanded manner as the supply situation becomes even more daunting and life on the waiting list becomes more uncertain and unproductive. Managed care could have a similar effect, although reliable data on effects to date are not available. Nevertheless, the success of managed care is based in part on a smaller and more efficient supply of services and stricter indications for medical interventions, which are conditions that may slow demand. Managed care is said also to be diminishing supply by less often carrying the care of seriously injured or ill patients to the point of potential donation using life support and other critical care interventions (L. Jacobbi, personal communication, July 17, 1997). It seems likely also that increased awareness of the cost of intensive care and increased familiarity with ethical issues surrounding end-of-life care may be having this effect in health care settings in general. If there are fewer declarations of brain death under managed (or conventional) care, this could tip the scales toward NHBDs and demand vigilance that these potential donations were actually obtained (Reiner, 1997). A similar incipient emphasis on NHBDs is suggested also by anecdotal reports that there may be increasing unwillingness of families to wait for brain death before discontinuing life support (Arnold, 1997).

A more promising alternative on the demand side lies in anticipated long-term advances coming from clinical experience and transplantation biology research. If these advances generate improvements in long-term organ survival, as they have in the past, they should shorten the waiting list and waiting times for various organs by eliminating or postponing the need for retransplantation. Patients awaiting the second transplant or more presently occupy about a fifth of the slots (mostly kidney) on the waiting list (UNOS, 1996). Reductions in demand would result from significant reductions in this category of patient, but only modest reductions are expected as graft survivals slowly improve.

IMPROVING SUPPLY

There is little optimism that procurement of organs from either living or brain-dead cadaver donors can be sharply accelerated, although marginal increases should be vigorously pursued. Living donor expansion will provide only one organ per donor and will not address the shortfall in organs that are not paired or transplantable in part. Also, each living donor incurs a risk of death or medical complication. Unpublicized mortality has reached "at least two dozen unpublished but certain donor deaths" (Sheil, 1995). Particularly in partial liver transplantation, the donor risk could be considered a real problem (Sterneck et al., 1995). However, advances in technology, such as laparoscopic nephrectomy, will reduce morbidity, may have a positive effect on mortality and, as reported anecdotally, may increase donation of kidneys from living donors. Increasing the pool of living donors through the use of genetically unrelated donors has raised a question for some that commercial considerations in organ procurement may be introduced if donors without spousal or strong friendship bonds are accepted (Hauptman and O'Connor, 1997). Nevertheless, an increase in living donors by primarily affecting the supply of kidneys affects the severest shortage and the largest category of transplants and helps patients with the longest waiting times.

Evans et al. (1992) have estimated the national, annual, potential number of brain-dead (heart-beating) donors at 6,900 to 10,700; the number of actual donors therefore is currently half this theoretical maximum and close to what one would expect if the upper-bound estimate of potential donors is correct, if all potential donors are approached (which is not the case), and if a traditional consent rate of 50% is achieved. Evans calculated an efficiency in U.S. organ procurement efforts in 1988–1989 from 37% to 59% (percentage of potential donors realized). A more recent study using 1990 data estimated 13,700 potential heart-beating donors, a nonidentification or failure-to-ask rate of 27%, and a consent rate of 45% of those asked (Gortmaker et al., 1996). These figures provide a somewhat lower assessment of efficiency. In either case, the supply of heart-beating donors does not appear sufficient to satisfy demand.

Current expanded donor criteria or acceptance of higher estimates, including NHBDs, by others (discussed below) (Bart et al., 1981; Nathan et al., 1991) may allow a potential that is greater than the accepted numbers for heart-beating donors. At the same time, seat belt, helmet, drunk driving, and gun safety laws and other public health measures as well as fear of HIV are said to be limiting the growth of or reducing the potential donor pool by lessening serious head trauma and disqualifying otherwise acceptable brain-dead donors (Arnold and Youngner, 1993; Evans et al., 1992). Increasing numbers of donors from the cerebrovascular or stroke category have maintained donor rates, although unfortunately at an older average age, in the face of these changes (UNOS, 1996).

A variously reported 13% to 28% of the population has filled out a donor card (Gallup, 1993; Martin and Meslin, 1994). Despite a combination of laws in the majority of states and rulings from both the Health Care Financing Administration and the Joint Commission on Accreditation of Healthcare Organizations that require essentially all hospitals to ask for donation, a quarter to a third of families of patients with appropriate medical status are never approached about donation and many potential donors are now being missed (Nathan et al., 1991; Siminoff et al., 1995). In addition, 20% of those with the diagnosis of brain death suffer cardiopulmonary arrest and death within 6 hours, and 50% within 24 hours, of admission to the intensive care unit. Thus, a very tight time schedule often frustrates efforts to complete necessary laboratory examinations and carry out other steps required to recover organs. Patients whose relatives were not asked about donation tend to be those who died sooner after admission and who did not die in the intensive care unit (Chapman et al., 1995). Lastly, as many as 35% of patients with very poor prognoses are not started on or are prematurely withdrawn from life support (Hibbard et al., 1992), and a recent survey disclosed that physicians did not recognize or declare brain death in 13% of potential donors, which eliminates the possibility of arranging donations in both situations (Wing and Chang, 1994).

In the past, the organ procurement effort in this country has been criticized for variable and sometimes very low productivity. In the context of a 1989 national rate of about 16 to 17 donors per million population (dmp),* some procurement organizations were achieving rates of about 2 dmp and others about 30 dmp. Other countries have improved procurement through better organization and work effort. Implementation in Spain of a unified, centralized program with an emphasis on improving coordination and performance was associated with a rapid increase from 19 to 28.5 dmp and an actual decrease in the waiting list in that country (Miranda, 1997). When assessing performance, it should be kept in

---

*Donors per million population refers only to cadaver donors (both heart-beating and non-heart-beating).

mind that local conditions other than procurement organization effectiveness—for example, public interest and understanding; local accident rates and trauma patterns; demographic, social, or cultural and religious factors; and possibly, the presence of local transplant services in the community—influence donor rates. Also, on an organization-specific basis, the number of donors is small and a particular year's donor rate may represent a statistical outlier rather than the usual performance.

Nevertheless, a UNOS model of supply and demand in liver procurement and transplantation using 1992 to 1994 data when national procurement numbers had improved to 19.2 dmp (range: 5.0 to 33.3 dmp) (Gortmaker et al., 1996), suggested that if organ procurement organizations' donation rates (for livers) could be raised to the level of the higher recovery OPOs (a potentially achievable level of 30 dmp each year and 80% average liver recovery per donor), this would represent about a 55% increase from the current national average, would cause a proportional decrease in waiting list deaths, and would dramatically reduce regional variations in waiting times (M. Ellison, personal communication, June 27, 1997). A rough approximation of equilibrium appeared within reach, provided there were no other changes on the supply or demand side, if effectiveness could be doubled. Caution should be used in drawing too many conclusions from these estimates, as noted earlier. Demand is unlikely to be stable as supply increases; different organs will have different equilibria; tissue-matching problems will affect the efficiency of kidney utilization; and categories of donor vary in their effectiveness in supplying organs. Nevertheless, the UNOS model does give a rough sense of the magnitude of the current problem and suggests a target that is theoretically not out of reach. Procurement in 1996 stood at 21 dmp nationally with a range of 7.1 to 37.4 dmp.

No rigorous cost-effectiveness analysis has been done to compare the costs and benefits of improving donor procurement. Each organ would require a separate analysis. Different cadaver donors have different efficiencies, ranging on average from 1.78 to 3.2 transplants each, and each transplant if successful takes a patient off dialysis or expensive treatment for organ failure. Of course, each transplant has its cost, and aside from kidney patients who can be maintained on dialysis, each patient who fails to get a transplant ultimately dies and eliminates all cost of any kind of care. Adding donors would generate additional cost (Evans, personal communication, 1997), although others disagree (UNOS, 1997), but a case could well be made for the cost-effectiveness of investing more in a stronger effort to improve organ donation and procurement rates. This assumes a reasonable balance between expenditures made and expenditures avoided, and the assignment of priority to relieving the human suffering, morbidity, and mortality associated with the present state of affairs.

Major improvements in the supply of organs could be made if the public consented to donation at rates higher than those currently experienced. Surveys show that the public consistently gives a high approval rating (85%) to the act of donation for organ transplantation (Gallup, 1993). Public willingness to donate personally or to consent, as a surrogate decision maker, to a family member's donation, runs from 45% to 50% and 53% to 68%, respectively (Evans, 1992). Gallup found even higher (69%) personal willingness to consider organ donation positively and 92% or 93% willingness to either honor a family member's wish to be a donor, if known, or give permission for donation as a surrogate decision maker, if unknown (Gallup, 1993).

However, the validity of these results has been questioned for a number of reasons, including the important one that a positive answer is the most socially acceptable answer. In Texas, during a time when applicants were required to make a personal decision in writing to obtain a driver's license, consent fell to 20% (Siminoff et al., 1995), and when permission to become a donor for a family member in a brain death situation is actually requested, consent varies from about 40% to 65% both in this country and abroad: 43.7% (Chapman et al., 1995), 46.5% (Siminoff et al., 1995), 50% (Hibbard et al., 1992), 57% (Morris et al., 1989), 62% (Nathan et al., 1991), and 65% (Kootstra, 1997); the U.S. average is about 50% (Braslow, 1997). Public concerns that a seriously ill or injured person known to have consented to organ donation may receive less aggressive care from physicians who are interested in organs for a potentially more promising or younger patient on the transplant waiting list are prominent among reasons for levels of consent that are so much lower than survey approval rates (Caplan, 1993). Some are also worried that organs may be removed before death has definitely occurred (Corlett, 1985). Of relevance to this concern, 21% of the public believes that a brain-dead person can recover from his or her injuries (Gallup, 1993).

At the actual time of request, families are emotionally traumatized. Decisions on transplantation may simply be more than they can handle in a crisis (Perkins, 1987), and the stress and confusion of fast-moving medical events may deny them adequate time to consider the merits of donation and resolve questions or misconceptions that are potential barriers to organ donation (Coolican, 1997; Gallup, 1993). Even after participating in the donation process, about half of donor families, particularly those who do not consent, report an incomplete understanding of brain death (Franz et al., 1997), and 10% to 15% report an inadequate general understanding and insufficient personal attention from transplant personnel (Pearson and Zurynski, 1995). Although evidence to direct and improve the request process suggests that discussions about brain death and discussions about organ donation should be decoupled, that private discussions are best, and that organ procurement organizations' (OPO) participation with hospital staff is advantageous, these methods are not uniformly understood or practiced (Beasley et al., 1997).

Understanding among the general public is undoubtedly less than that reported for donor families, which suggests a need for more and better educational as well as recruitment efforts. A significant minority of the public holds one or more misconceptions—for example, that donation is deforming or is not possible over age 55 (Gallup, 1993). On the other hand, some have expressed skepticism about the effect of periodic donor campaigns that lack the resources to maintain the intensity necessary to have more than a minimal effect on public understanding and opinion. They have noted that the resources devoted to public education at the organ procurement level averaged only $158,000 per year per organization in 1994 (L. Jacobbi, personal communication, July 17, 1997). This argues for devoting greater resources in general to public education. More specifically, those groups most likely to be responsive could be targeted with carefully focused information. Those involved in deciding about donation could be educated at the time of the decision through making a greater investment in trained, coordinated, and monitored procurement personnel; better-informed medical professionals; and well-planned and directed donor recruitment procedures (Partnership for Organ Donation, unpublished work, June 1997; Perkins, 1987; Siminoff et al., 1995). Reports indicate plenty of room for improvement here (Franz et al., 1997).

Continuing efforts to improve donation within the current structure of the transplantation effort are important. In view of the factors discussed, it is reasonable to assume that real increases in procurement of organs from currently accepted donor categories could be achieved through: better preparation of the public for the eventuality of being confronted with a loved one's death and the possibility of becoming an organ donor; appropriate discussions with potential donors; expanded criteria for cadaver donor acceptance; improved public and professional education; higher request and consent percentages; and expanded governmental and legislative initiatives. Work is needed in all the areas noted above. A number of other helpful suggestions have also been made (Riether and Mahler, 1995), and an array of more recent efforts holds promise. These include legislation establishing a donor registry linked to driver's license renewal in Illinois that does not force a yes or no on donation as was previously the case in Texas, but rather indicates interest in potentially being a donor. This registry has achieved a 38% positive response and is associated with a 52% increase in donors at the Regional Organ Bank of Illinois. An associated intense public campaign has played a key role in this result also (Anderson, personal communication, 1997). In 1994, Pennsylvania enacted legislation that requires routine notification to OPOs of all hospital deaths and places OPO staff in control of requesting consent for organ donation. This legislation also includes penalties for noncompliance. The program has been associated with a 32% increase in transplants from the Delaware Valley (Pennsylvania) Transplant Program. Most recently, New York has enacted similar legislation, but without the noncompliance penalties. Arizona provides an example of a state that repealed presumed donor consent on the driver's license and enacted legislation that statutorily confirms the primacy of advance directives, requires specific training for personnel seeking consent for donation, and requires only distribution of a donor card and a red "donor" sticker at application for a driver's license (L. Futral, personal communication, September 17, 1997). The nationally active Coalition on Donation has generated more than $30 million in donated media time and space in the few years since it was established and, with bipartisan congressional support, generated donor cards that were inserted in 70 million income tax refunds in 1997. A new organization, the Redford Institute for Transplant Awareness, using its access to the media and the entertainment industry, is also beginning campaigns.

Current levels of effort including recent positive developments may have a significant effect and, along with further efforts, should be vigorously followed up. Alone, however, they seem unlikely to provide multiple marginal improvements of the magnitude necessary to resolve the demand crisis. The number of variables and the lack of quantitative information that have been cited preclude any certainty about supply and demand. Real demand seems likely to be many times the supply possible with current scenarios. Therefore, transplant programs are being challenged, particularly since the Pittsburgh protocol in 1992 (Arnold, 1995; DeVita and Snyder, 1993), to explore whether a new category of donor, the non-heart-beating donor, might add significantly to supply, although this kind of donor is more a refinement of one of the earliest categories that had fallen into relative disuse than a new concept.

3

Background

THE HISTORICAL NHBD

After unsuccessful attempts at solid organ transplantation in the early 1950s, the successful transplantation of a kidney from one identical twin to the other in 1954 reassured scientists that the actual technical transfer of a major functioning solid organ from one person to another was a practical possibility. The biological and immunological problems that remained were at least in part identified, if by no means fully understood or resolved. The success of a kidney transplant between fraternal twins in 1959 suggested that these were not insurmountable either, and indeed, existing and subsequently developed drugs mitigated the effects of the immune response, delaying or preventing rejection of the transplanted organ. The development of immunological tests, including tissue typing and matching, also played a role in improving results. Experimental transplant programs started with kidney transplantation, to which were added liver (1963) and heart (1967) transplantation along with pancreas, lung, various combinations such as kidney-pancreas and heart-lung, and more recently intestine (DeVita et al., 1993; Federle, 1995; Starzl and Demetris, 1995).

Early transplant programs obtained organs either from healthy, living, related donors or from cadaver donors. These cadaver donors were declared dead by cardiopulmonary criteria. A determination of death by neurologic criteria, although a legal option in the sense that state laws allowed physicians to make determinations of death according to their own practice and custom, was not generally accepted. Physicians of the time were reluctant to pronounce death in a patient who had continued heart function. Such cadaver donors provided kidneys most commonly, although there were some successful attempts to transplant other solid organs.

Kidneys, as the primary organs recovered from these cadavers, generally had been exposed for a considerable period of time (by today's standards) to failing circulation and did not approach the ideal—perfusion with warm, oxygenated blood up to the time of removal from the donor. Results were understandably below current expectations. Somewhat damaged kidneys suffered frequently from delayed function in the recipient, as is observed particularly in NHBD kidneys today. Such kidneys experience acute rejection more often and have poorer long-term survivals (Troppmann et al., 1996). Nevertheless, early versions of organ perfusion and preservation technologies similar to those currently in use were developed, and transplantation using these (uncontrolled) NHBDs continued to be pursued in Japanese and some European centers (Anaise and Rapaport, 1993).

NEUROLOGIC CRITERIA FOR DEATH

In 1968, the Harvard neurologic definition and criteria for death were published (Report of the Ad Hoc Committee of the Harvard Medical School, 1968). These essentially amounted to total unresponsiveness and loss of the brain's integrative control of body physiology as measured by various clinical and technical tests. Over the next few years, a model definition of death based on irreversible loss of function of the whole brain including the brain stem, or irreversible cessation of cardiopulmonary function, was enacted widely into state law, enabling the recovery of organs from "brain-dead" cadavers who maintained breathing and circulation on artificial ventilation. Organs recovered from these donors were viable and were more likely to function well immediately and to yield good long-term results. As a result, the original approach of recovering organs from NHBDs gradually ceased to be a significant part of transplantation in the United States and many Western countries.

Brain death is now legally and ethically accepted in every state. However, there are still some misconceptions about the whole-brain determination of death, for example: (1) many practitioners do not know and do not practice the correct determination of brain death (Mejia and Pollack, 1995); (2) some varying technical signs of brain function often persist in brain-dead patients (Halevy and Brody, 1993); (3) physicians and others often speak in ways that imply that there is brain death and then real death when heart and lung function is lost, and they use the time of the latter as the time of death for death certificates; (4) surveys and questionnaires indicate that about a third of physicians, some donor families, and certainly many in the general public do not really understand the concept of brain death (Gallup, 1993; Youngner et al., 1989); and (5) it is difficult for many to consider a donor dead whose heart is still beating and whose respiration continues, even though circulation and other normal body functions can be maintained only artificially and with difficulty (Arnold and Youngner,

1993; Field et al., 1988; Parisi et al., 1982). Nevertheless, despite these conceptual difficulties, the use of brain-dead (heart-beating) donors has been widely accepted at present in the United States and is the basis for a part of the improved results of transplantation.*

---

*Acceptance of the concept of brain death is not universal. There are rare, spirited objections (McMahan, 1995).

4

The Modern Non-Heart-Beating Donor

THE CONTROLLED NHBD

More than 50,000 patients are on the waiting list for organs in this country (UNOS, 1997), awaiting a lifesaving treatment for which personnel, facilities, and for the insured, funds are not limiting. The waiting list not only is growing rapidly but likely is a significant undercount, omitting many, as noted, who withdraw or who are discouraged by the long waits and uncertain prospects. Waiting list deaths are also mounting, and they too may be underestimated because deaths of those removed from the list as they deteriorate beyond transplantability are not counted as waiting list deaths. In reaction to the increasing need for organs, transplant programs have begun to revisit the traditional sources of donors, focusing on the controlled category of NHBDs, although some, such as the University of Wisconsin at Madison, have always had an active NHBD program. The Pittsburgh "Policy for the Management of Terminally Ill Patients Who May Become Organ Donors After Death" (Arnold, 1995), devised after extensive local review and subject to wide commentary from the ethics and medical community after issuance, was emblematic of this return to former sources. Some of the issues raised by the Pittsburgh protocol, examined by the medical and ethics communities and reported in depth in the medical and ethics literature, have not been conclusively resolved and are taken up again in this report.

As noted earlier, the NHBD is a donor whose death is defined by "irreversible cessation of circulatory and respiratory functions" as opposed to "irreversible cessation of all functions of the entire brain, including the brainstem" (Uniform Determination of Death Act, 12 Uniform Laws Annotated 320 [1990 Suppl.]). Organs recovered from such a donor cannot be ideally suited for transplantation because cardiopulmonary death means that organs will not continue to receive oxygenated blood up to the moment of removal from the donor. Before the establishment of the whole-brain determination of death, NHBDs were the only kind of cadaver donor, but the essentially total phasing out of the NHBD thereafter is convincing testimony to the preferability of organs from brain-dead (heart-beating) donors. In fact, in the transplantation literature, discussions of a return to the practice of procuring organs from NHBDs almost invariably begin by explaining that the shortage of organs and the intense pressure to increase supply are driving consideration of organs retrieved from NHBDs (Bos, 1995).

The modern, controlled NHBD differs in a number of ways from the historical, uncontrolled NHBD. Over the past several decades, court cases, ethical debates, public reporting, major religious pronouncements, and undoubtedly the mere passage of time have allowed better public understanding and acceptance and an alleviation of concerns about withdrawal of life-sustaining treatment from certain patients (Banks, 1995; Council on Scientific Affairs and Council on Ethical and Judicial Affairs of the American Medical Association, 1990; Emanuel, 1988; *Kennedy Institute of Ethics Journal,* 1993; President's Commission, 1983). These patients are either competent with intolerable quality of life or incompetent, but not brain dead, because of severe, generally neurological, illness or injury with an extremely poor prognosis as to survival or any meaningful functional status. A significant number of patients, therefore, can be identified for whom, after proper safeguards and with informed consent from the competent patient or from surrogate decision maker(s) for the incompetent patient, life-sustaining treatment may be discontinued. These patients who are being maintained on artificial ventilation or, occasionally, circulatory assistance will suffer irreversible cessation of circulatory and respiratory functions within a short interval after withdrawal of support. Death will almost always occur soon enough after withdrawal of support to allow the removal of viable organs for transplantation.

This kind of NHBD—the controlled NHBD—is the one that most closely simulates the ideal conditions for organ recovery which exist with organs procured from heart-beating cadaver donors; that is, it is the donor with the shortest time between absence of circulation and removal of organs, and it is the most common kind of NHBD in the United States. These donors are controlled because the timing and thus the process of donation are controlled through the timing of life support. The time interval for organ recovery starts with the withdrawal of life support and ends usually within 1 or 2 hours. Under certain circumstances and in some programs a different interval may be selected if the patient dies within that time. If the patient's death after withdrawal of support is delayed beyond an hour or two, a determination is often made that organ viability has suffered too much during the dying process to warrant transplantation.

> **Box 4.1**
> **Maastricht Categories for Non-Heart-Beating Donors**
>
> I. Dead on arrival.
> II. Unsuccessful resuscitation.
> III. Awaiting cardiac death.
> IV. Cardiac death in a brain-dead donor.
>
> SOURCE: Kootstra, 1995.

THE UNCONTROLLED NHBD

There are a number of other categories of NHBDs, referred to as uncontrolled. Some, primarily Europeans, separate NHBDs into numbered categories (See Box 4.1) including three uncontrolled donor categories (Maastricht categories I, II, and IV) and one controlled donor category (Maastricht III) (Kootstra, 1995). Uncontrolled NHBDs include those whose hearts have stopped shortly before arrival at the hospital (category I), those who suffer cardiopulmonary arrest in the hospital and cannot be resuscitated (category II), and those who, having been determined brain dead, suffer unexpected cardiac arrest (category IV). Uncontrolled donors make up the bulk of many European programs. Some American programs consider both categories III and IV as controlled (see chapter 5, J. Light, personal communication, 1997). Kidneys, livers, pancreases, and lungs can be recovered from controlled NHBDs (D'Alessandro et al., 1995a,b). Recovery of other than kidneys is problematic from uncontrolled donors (Kootstra, 1997) but may be possible with early organ perfusion using the appropriate cold solutions. Often this intervention must be started so quickly after death that circumstances do not allow consent to be obtained, which poses a problem in the United States. The contribution of kidneys retrieved from uncontrolled NHBDs to the kidney supply is fortunate because this is the organ most in demand (D'Alessandro et al., 1995a; Kootstra, 1997). On the other hand, in terms of addressing the supply shortage, it is unfortunate that uncontrolled donors with their limitations are potentially the largest category of donors (Light et al., 1996; Nicholson, 1996). Furthermore, in all types of NHBDs, organ recovery and transplantation rates are lower than in heart-beating donors, as previously noted.

Of the various types of NHBDs, it is clear that the uncontrolled donor has the greatest interval between cessation of circulatory function and cold perfusion or removal of organs. During this time, which in some programs may exceed an hour, there is deterioration of all organs. In the case of kidneys, this means delay of graft function in as many as 60% (Kootstra, 1997), 74%

(Hoshinaga et al., 1995), or even 100% of cases (Nicholson et al., 1997; Varty et al., 1994). This compares to the 22% to 26% reported achievable in controlled NHBD programs (A.M. D'Alessandro, personal communication, July 21, 1997; Orloff et al., 1994). The best figures are in brain-dead (heart-beating) or living donors, averaging around 20%, although some programs using machine perfusion achieve 7% to 8% (A. M. D'Alessandro, personal communication, July 21, 1997). Delayed graft function does not prohibit kidney transplantation because function can be replaced by dialysis until recovery. Other organs are less tolerant of circulatory arrest and without artificial functional substitutes are said to be effectively ruled out (Kootstra, 1997), although this situation may change. Delayed kidney function is also associated with decreased long-term (3-year) graft survival (UNOS, 1997, Report of Center Specific Graft and Survival Rates) and with more frequent acute rejection reactions (Wijnen et al., 1995). Ultimately, this combination of delayed function and acute rejection is also associated with decreased long-term graft survival (Cosio et al., 1997; Troppmann et al., 1996).

For all kinds of NHBDs, these conditions have generated intense pressure to approach the favorable conditions of the brain-dead (heart-beating) and living donor. This requires the following, to the extent possible: a precise prediction of the timing of, and a short interval to, death; a prompt determination of death and organ retrieval; a rapid initiation of cold preservation; and an acceptance of a full array of interventions that might enhance organ viability and stabilize the patient for donation. These are the kinds of pressures that have justified "presumed consent" laws in many countries, which authorize, unless there is notice to the contrary, nonconsensual organ perfusion or even in some cases organ removal while awaiting consent for donation (Veatch and Pitt, 1995). In the United States, the District of Columbia has a law that allows perfusion and cooling without consent and a successful program that utilizes this statutory authority to procure uncontrolled NHBDs (87 Stat. 813:D.C. Code § 1-233(c)(1)). Virginia and Florida also have such a law, although in Florida no nonconsensual cooling is done despite statutory authority (Reiner, 1997). A few states have proposed but not enacted similar laws—the Regional Organ Bank of Illinois practiced nonconsensual cooling for a short time (UNOS, 1996)—and a number of observers have urged a policy of initiating cooling without consent (Anaise and Rapaport, 1993).

CURRENT STATUS OF THE NHBD IN TRANSPLANTATION

The exploration of the modern NHBD, in an attempt to redress the imbalance between supply and demand, began in the early 1990s, and was enhanced by the far-reaching discussion and analysis of the 1992 Pittsburgh protocol. Actual transplantation using controlled NHBDs in the United States started as a small effort and has remained so. Figures cited in one report (DeVita, 1995) were 20 total NHBDs in 1992 and 45 total NHBDs, of which 34 were controlled, in 1993. UNOS data (M. Ellison, personal communication, June 27, 1997) in Tables 4.1A and 4.1B suggest a baseline of a small number of uncontrolled NHBDs.

TABLE 4.1A. Non-Heart-Beating Donors Recovered in the United States: 1993–1996

Year	No. of Donors Recovered	Percentage of Organ-Specific Donors				
		Kidney	Liver	Heart	Lung	Pancreas
1993	43	100.0	37.2	4.7	9.3	19.4
1994	59	98.3	39.0	8.5	10.2	13.6
1995	44	100.0	22.7	0.0	4.5	4.5
1996	65	96.9	24.6	0.0	1.5	10.8
1993–1996, Overall	211	98.6	30.8	3.3	6.1	11.4

SOURCE: Based on UNOS OPTN/Scientific Registry data as of June 14, 1997. Data subject to change based on future data submissions.

TABLE 4.1B. Number of Transplants Performed with Non-Heart-Beating Donors: 1993–1996 Controlled vs. Not Controlled

Organ	Category	Year of Transplant				1993–1996, Overall
		1993	1994	1995	1996	
Kidney	Controlled	0	21	48	67	136
	Not controlled	68	63	23	28	182
Liver	Controlled	0	5	3	9	17
	Not controlled	9	7	3	2	21
Heart	Controlled	0	0	0	0	0
	Not controlled	0	2	0	0	2
Pancreas	Controlled	0	0	1	6	7
	Not controlled	5	0	0	1	6
Lung	Controlled	0	0	0	2	2
	Not controlled	1	0	0	0	1
Total	Controlled	0	26	52	84	162
	Not controlled	83	72	26	31	212
Overall		83	98	78	115	374

SOURCE: Based on UNOS OPTN/Scientific Registry data as of June 14, 1997. Data subject to change based on future data submissions.

Given the lack of data and the reporting of controlled and uncontrolled numbers together in 1993 and part of 1994 (reported as "not controlled"), little can be concluded about uncontrolled NHBD trends, but the numbers appear fairly stable. The small number of controlled NHBD transplants may be slowly increasing, although here too it is early to draw firm conclusions. The overwhelming majority of these NHBD transplants (85%) were kidneys, as is the case in other countries; and low transplant or donor rates seem consistent over time. Roughly half of transplant programs (120) and organ procurement organizations (36) recovered organs from at least one NHBD during 1993–1996.

TABLE 4.2. Kaplan–Meier Graft Survival Rates for Transplants Performed 1993–1995, Controlled vs. Not Controlled for Non-Heart-Beating Donors

Cadaveric Organ	Non-Heart-Beating Donor	Controlled[a]	Months Post-transplant	n	Survival Rate[b]	Standard Error
Kidney	Yes	Yes	6	63	88.1	4.0
			12	45	86.4	4.0
		No	6	149	81.6	3.1
			12	138	78.9	3.3
			18	123	78.1	3.4
			24	106	76.3	3.5
	No		6	23,262	87.6	0.2
			12	19,877	85.0	0.2
			18	16,091	82.8	0.3
			24	13,123	80.7	0.3
Liver	Yes	Yes	6	7	—	—
			12	7	—	—
			18	6	—	—
			24	6	—	—
		No	6	18	46.8	11.6
			12	17	40.9	11.5
			18	16	32.7	11.8
			24	15	32.7	11.8
	No		6	9,551	79.0	0.4
			12	7,823	75.2	0.4
			18	6,339	72.1	0.5
			24	5,311	70.0	0.5

[a] Data on controlled versus not controlled were not collected prior to April 1994.
[b] "—" means that a survival rate could not be computed because n at risk is less than 10.
SOURCE: Based on UNOS OPTN/Scientific Registry data as of June 14, 1997. Data subject to correction based on future data submission or correction.

The results of transplantation reported since 1994, the first year that UNOS began keeping separate statistics on controlled and uncontrolled NHBDs, are shown in Table 4.2, which, because of small numbers, includes only kidney and liver data. The same data are displayed in Table 4.3, except that results of transplants using organs from NHBDs are reported in total rather than separately as controlled and uncontrolled. These data are consistent with the conclusion that transplants using kidneys from NHBDs (primarily controlled NHBDs) provide results close to or almost as good as brain-dead (heart-beating) donors. In Table 4.3 total results of liver transplants using NHBD livers are dramatically worse than liver heart-beating donor results, and since uncontrolled NHBD liver results in Table 4.2 are slightly better than total results, a small group of more successful controlled donor grafts is not hidden in the total. Because of insufficient numbers, these data are preliminary indications only, but they tend to support the promise of NHBD kidney transplantation, perhaps with slightly reduced graft survivals; to confirm that fewer organs per donor are recovered from NHBDs, and these are mostly kidneys; and to suggest that further improvements in liver transplantation with NHBD livers could, and probably will be achieved. They are also consistent with reports from elsewhere, except that controlled NHBD liver transplants, reported separately, have much higher success rates (Casavilla et al., 1995a,b; D'Alessandro et al., 1995a,b). A separate analysis using UNOS data of 204 kidney transplants supports these conclusions (Cho et al., unpublished work, 1997).

TABLE 4.3. Kaplan–Meier Graft Survival Rates for Transplants Performed 1993–1995

Cadaveric Organ	Non-Heart-Beating Donor	Months Post-transplant	n	Survival Rate	Standard Error
Kidney	Yes	6	212	83.6	2.5
		12	183	81.2	2.7
		18	149	79.8	2.8
		24	125	78.3	2.9
	No	6	23,262	87.6	0.2
		12	19,877	85.0	0.2
		18	16,091	82.8	0.3
		24	13,123	80.7	0.3
Liver	Yes	6	25	43.7	9.7
		12	24	39.3	9.6
		18	22	26.2	9.9
		24	21	26.2	9.9
	No	6	9,551	79.0	0.4
		12	7,823	75.2	0.4
		18	6,339	72.1	0.5
		24	5,311	70.0	0.5

SOURCE: Based on UNOS OPTN/Scientific Registry data as of June 14, 1997. Data subject to correction based on future data submission or correction.

Reports from individual programs in this country and abroad comparing results of transplants using organs from controlled and uncontrolled NHBDs with brain-dead (heart-beating) or living donors have generally documented competitive 1-year kidney graft survivals but provided less information on longer-term function. Some longer-term results have been encouraging (Alvarez-Rodriguez et al., 1995; Schlumpf et al., 1996; Wijnen et al., 1995); whereas others are less so (Andrews et al., 1995; Nicholson, 1996; Nicholson et al., 1997; Phillips et al., 1994; Szostek et al., 1995; Valero et al., 1995). Rates of delayed kidney graft function have been high, particularly in transplants using organs from uncontrolled NHBDs, as noted earlier. These results should be compared both to results from the best types of donors and to the hazards and the economic and human costs endured by patients on the waiting list or by the set of patients who because of implicit rationing are not formally listed. Many observers have concluded that they support aggressive continued development and use of organs from NHBDs as a resource for kidney transplantation and, especially with controlled and perhaps with uncontrolled donors, for other organs as well. All this depends of course on the availability of reasonable numbers of such donors.

The numbers of NHBD organ transplants in the United States cannot have had any significant effect in meeting demand to date. From 1993 to 1996, NHBDs made up around 1% of total cadaver donors, varying between 0.8% (1995) and 1.2% (1994, 1996) (M. Ellison, personal communication, June 27, 1997). Meanwhile, European programs (Kootstra and Daemen, 1995) have reported as much as a 40% expansion in cadaver donors (mostly uncontrolled NHBDs) (Daemen et al., 1996), and a 20% to 25% increase is routinely achieved or predicted (Nicholson et al., 1997; Wijnen et al., 1995). One large program in this country reports that 16 NHBDs (all controlled) comprised 12.3% of total cadaver donors (a 14% expansion) and 8.6% of transplanted organs during a 17-month interval in 1993 and 1994 (D'Alessandro et al., 1995b). A second program reports 26 NHBDs (12 controlled) during a 5.5-year period leading up to 1995 (Casavilla et al., 1995a). One U.S. source (Nathan et al., 1991) estimated that controlled NHBDs have the potential to increase cadaver donors by at least 25%. More expansive estimates have also been made for a more inclusive group of NHBDs: 25,000–26,000 NHBDs, 123 dmp (Nathan, 1997) as cited in Daemen et al. (1996), 2.3% of hospital deaths (Bart et al., 1981); the number of uncontrolled NHBDs being six times greater than the number of controlled NHBDs (Light et al., 1994).

If the estimates are close to accurate, organs recovered from at least 1,000 controlled NHBDs could be added to the cadaver donor organ supply each year, and probably more. When added to potential increases in the supply of organs from living and heart-beating donors, this would have substantial impact. Yet at best, only 6% to 7% of this number is being reached. Significant realization of estimated uncontrolled NHBD potential would have an even greater effect. Of course, these estimates are speculative.

In 1994, a survey showed that 20 of 66 OPOs (30%) had NHBD protocols; of the 66 OPOs, 25 had procured and 23 had transplanted organs from NHBDs (UNOS, 1994). In 1997, the Institute of Medicine (IOM) asked all (at that time)

63 OPOs to submit their NHBD protocols as part of the information gathered for this report. Information was collected from 100%. Some protocols under development were not submitted, but all final approved versions were obtained (see chapter 5). Slightly more than half of OPOs had protocols, although a larger proportion reported that they were actually recovering organs from such donors. Other OPOs had a number of reasons for not exploring recovery of organs from NHBDs, as described later. In fact, the majority of transplant programs served by OPOs do not perform transplants from NHBDs (M. Ellison, personal communication, June 27, 1997), and some programs limit their efforts to controlled donors, which also limits the amount of expansion that is possible (D'Alessandro, 1995a).

Given a social consensus, there are a number of things that could improve the supply of organs relative to demand. Steps to improve the supply of organs from one category of donor often improve those of other categories as well. Steps that might be taken include the following: investments in improving rapid responsiveness of hospitals to identify potential donors, development and implementation of better public education and of better ways to get consent for donation, uniformly asking for consent, better support of donors (e.g., better early recognition and better initiation of life support and maintenance), wider acceptance of expanded donor criteria including emotionally related living donors, more organs retrieved per donor, research to improve organ use (e.g., screening methods for viability to enhance use of good organs and minimize use of organs that are not in good condition), increased research in general to improve transplantation success rates and reduce retransplantation, and continued experiments at the state and ultimately, national level, (e.g., registries, required notification of hospital deaths to OPOs, or perhaps extension of required requests to potential category III NHBDs). This list should also include the following: expansion of the procurement of controlled and uncontrolled NHBDs, improved effectiveness of OPOs and OPO policy, and procedural readiness to access all categories of donors. This report also makes recommendations that could provide a more consistent, publicly acceptable nationwide NHBD effort, which could have a positive effect on donation rates.

There are both scientific justification and historical precedent for expanding into the NHBD category, and a substantial increase* in donors seems quite possible as a result. Given the uncertain assumptions and the variable existing predictions involved, an estimate of the magnitude of the increase would be highly speculative. In view of the shortfall in organ supply and its human cost, how-

---

*As noted earlier, the size of any increase is speculative, but credible experts (Nathan, 1991) and transplanters (Kootstra, 1997) have estimated upward of 25% more cadaver donors. Safar (1988) has estimated that there are annually 250,000 acute, presenile, not incurably diseased cases of death in the United States in which resuscitation attempts might be justified. Recovery of organs from even a small fraction of these potential uncontrolled NHBDs would represent a substantial contribution.

ever, best efforts should be made to develop reasonable solutions. At the same time, there should be a realistic understanding of the limitations of the NHBD given current technology and procedures. Both the lower numbers of organs per donor (because of their deterioration in the body of the donor) and the condition of the organs that are recovered limit the benefits, and undoubtedly increase the costs of NHBDs relative to other categories of donors. There also seems to be considerable inertia in developing procurement policies, as well as uncertainty and anxiety about the proper policies and procedures to adopt. In some OPOs, there is opposition to NHBDs, and because some of this opposition is said to reflect public concerns, it could be difficult to change. Identification, discussion, and if possible, resolution of some of the outstanding issues concerning the proper ethical and medical management of these donors might help to overcome this uncertainty or opposition if they are indeed among the reasons for the very slow expansion of the NHBD pool.

5

Survey of Organ Procurement Organization and Transplant Program Policies

The National Organ Transplantation Act of 1984 (NOTA) established the national Organ Procurement and Transplantation Network (OPTN) to coordinate organ sharing among transplant centers in the United States. The United Network for Organ Sharing, which was incorporated in 1984, is a private entity composed of individual transplant centers and organizations responsible for obtaining organs from donors and allocating and distributing organs to recipients within the United States. UNOS was given the contract by the Division of Transplantation of the Department of Health and Human Services (DHHS) to oversee and maintain the OPTN in 1986. This contract assigns UNOS responsibility for developing organ allocation policies and includes a limited number of specific projects to increase the supply of organs. UNOS also oversees the recipient waiting list, collects information on donors, and maintains the Scientific Registry, which tracks recipient data after transplantation.

According to UNOS, its role is "to establish a national Organ Procurement and Transplantation Network under the Public Health and Safety Act, in order to improve the effectiveness of the nation's renal and extrarenal organ procurement, distribution, and transplantation systems by increasing the availability of, and access to, donor organs for patients with end-stage organ failure; to develop, implement, and maintain quality assurance activities; and to systematically gather and analyze data and regularly publish the results of the national experience in organ procurement" (UNOS Articles of Incorporation).

Organ procurement organizations, as established under NOTA, must belong to the OPTN and report data to the Scientific Registry. Each OPO orchestrates and oversees the organ donation process at one or more transplant centers. OPOs are responsible for organ quality including appropriate preservation and packaging and assurance that adequate material for tissue typing is procured, divided, and packaged (UNOS Policies as of March 7, 1997). OPOs also act as liaisons between individual hospitals and UNOS. Eligibility for reimbursement under Medicare requires that transplant centers be members of the OPTN. OPOs are responsible for identifying, evaluating, and maintaining the donor; obtaining consent from the patient or patient's family for the removal of organs; verifying pronouncement of death; and ensuring that information about the donor is entered into the UNOS national computer system, and that the approved UNOS organ allocation program is executed for each donor organ.

INTEREST IN OPO NHBD PROTOCOLS

All 63 organ procurement organizations in the United States were identified by UNOS for an IOM survey of their NHBD protocols, carried out in May, June, and July 1997, which simply asked for a copy of OPO NHBD protocols and followed up all nonresponders to obtain a protocol or to confirm the absence of a protocol and elicit reasons for such an absence. (See Appendix C for the request letter, a listing of the OPOs, and a map.) Protocols were evaluated as described below using a checklist including: approved; draft; for controlled NHBDs; for uncontrolled NHBDs; cannula use; determination of death; use of heparin and regitine; OPO referral, life support withdrawal decisionmaking, and donation discussions; and family contacts and location of withdrawal. Additional anecdotal information elicited during telephone follow-ups is included when judged to be worthwhile. The survey was performed to provide a basis of information on actual NHBD procurement practices. This information assisted in the analysis and preparation of conclusions and recommendations on issues identified earlier in this report. Fifty-four of the surveyed OPOs are independent. Nine are located in specific hospitals. According to UNOS data, 20 donor hospitals and OPOs recovered organs from NHBDs in 1996, and 36 recovered organs from NHBDs from 1993 to 1996.

PROTOCOL STATISTICS

All of the OPOs responded to the IOM request for a copy of their NHBD protocols, either by mail or via phone interview. Twenty-five OPOs have approved NHBD protocols in effect. Nine OPOs reported that they were in the process of drafting, approving, or reevaluating their NHBD protocols. A few OPOs reported that their NHBD protocols were being reevaluated by medical and ethics committees after the recent adverse national publicity and other negative reactions.

ORGAN PROCUREMENT AND TRANSPLANT PROGRAM POLICIES

Twenty-nine OPOs indicated that they did not have an NHBD protocol, were not actively engaged in developing one, and did not recover organs from NHBDs. Explanations given for the absence of an NHBD protocol and program included lack of member hospital interest (OPOs have no jurisdiction over hospitals in this regard); lack of equipment; lack of a sufficient population in the OPO area; desire to focus on heart-beating (brain-dead) donors; inability of the OPO and hospitals to resolve concerns regarding NHBDs; fear of negative media coverage; community opposition; and potential for less viable organs from NHBDs. Many of the OPOs without NHBD protocols expressed an interest in learning more about the issues surrounding NHBD procedures and hearing the findings of this report.

The IOM received a total of 29 NHBD protocols from various OPOs (25 approved, 4 in draft form or in the approval process). Twenty-four protocols are limited to controlled NHBD organ procurement. Five protocols cover both controlled and uncontrolled NHBDs, although in one of these the coverage of uncontrolled NHBDs includes only category IV (a category where the distinction between controlled and uncontrolled is somewhat vague in this country). The following analysis pertains only to controlled NHBDs unless otherwise noted. This analysis also includes information from protocols currently in draft form, which are subject to change. Nevertheless, both the approved and the draft protocols received and reviewed by the IOM reflect current thinking regarding NHBDs. Areas of important procedural differences exist among protocols beyond what might be expected as reflecting the local needs and concerns of regional hospitals and OPOs. These include variation in the involvement of an OPO in approaching the family for consent for donation, OPO interventions and preparation of the donor prior to death, medications administered prior to death, and criteria for the determination of death once life support has been withdrawn. Some hospitals have different NHBD provisions than the OPO, and some protocols are really those of the sole NHBD transplant center covered by the OPO.

IDENTIFICATION OF POTENTIAL DONORS

Each protocol begins with an identification of and criteria for potential NHBD candidates. Most describe the conditions for a potential NHBD as a "patient (who) has severe head injury but does not meet brain death criteria, and is ventilator dependent." Thereafter, however, the sequence of events for contacting OPOs, securing consent from families, and assessing donor suitability varies among protocols. Some differences simply reflect procedural preferences, but others appear to reflect ethical differences.

A majority of protocols set limits for the age of NHBDs. Most require donors to be between 5 and 55 years of age. The narrowest age range is infant to age 35, and the widest, newborn to age 80. Most protocols also stipulate that the potential NHBD must have a known cause of death, not be classified as high-risk by the Centers for Disease Control and Prevention (CDC) (intravenous [IV] drug users, homosexual or bisexual males, HIV positive status, etc.), and have no known history of hypertension, sepsis, or cancer except for primary brain tumors.

All protocols emphasize that the medical evaluation of the donor by the physician prior to decisions to withdraw life support shall not be influenced by the possibility of donation. The policy of drawing a strict line between patient and donor is present in each. However, the protocol for implementing and safeguarding this policy varies greatly among OPOs. Candidates for organ donation are identified based on evaluation of their medical records and clinical data. Five NHBD protocols specify notification about such potential donors to the OPO before the decision to withdraw life support has been made by the family and physician. Most OPOs are contacted only after the decision to withdraw support has been made and before the option of donation is presented and discussed with families. Routine referral of dying patients to the OPO, pursuant either to state law or to hospital-OPO policy, undoubtedly introduces donation as a possibility in the course of care of terminal patients, as discussed in the following sections of this chapter.

Four OPOs begin evaluating and testing the donor for suitability (including clinical evaluation, medical history review, and laboratory tests) before the decision to withdraw life support has been made, and about half of the OPOs begin clinical evaluation before obtaining consent for donation. A few protocols describe discussion among attending physicians and transplant surgeons before the decision to withdraw life support, and a large majority before decisions to donate. One protocol states that the "OPO representative will discuss the possibility of procurement with the attending physician to ensure that the physician agrees with termination of support on medical grounds" before the decision to terminate support is made.

Many OPO protocols outline the tests and procedures for determining donor suitability. An apnea test to reveal how dependent the patient is upon a ventilator is often used to determine whether the patient will die relatively quickly after withdrawal of life support. One detailed evaluation specifies the laboratory and diagnostic tests, serology tests, blood specimens for tissue typing, and apnea tests that should be performed to evaluate the donor. Other protocols are less technical and do not detail the tests to be performed: "potential donor meets OPO standard medical criteria for donation." Five OPO protocols restrict the type of organs that can be procured from NHBDs to kidney or liver and kidney (other organs may be used for research) due to concern about damage to other organs caused by time without circulation.

APPROACH TO FAMILY FOR CONSENT

All OPO protocols explicitly require that discussion of donation and the informed consent process with the patient or family take place only after a decision to withdraw life support has been made. The protocols have different views on who should initiate discussion of donation with family members. A few prefer that the attending physician initiate this discussion. If the family expresses interest, OPO coordinators are then contacted for further explanation and discussion of the donation process. Other protocols do not require attending physician involvement and indicate that the "option to donate shall be presented to the family by the OPO transplant coordinator." Still other protocols emphasize the collective presence and cooperation of the attending physician, OPO coordinator, hospital witness, and patient advocate during discussions of donation with families. These provisions are interesting given the increasing body of state legislation and reporting in the medical literature requiring or strongly suggesting that trained and experienced personnel participate in donation discussions.

One protocol allows donation only if the interest in organ donation is initiated by the family of the patient: "NHBD will never be offered as an option for any patient by a member of the health care team, transplant team, OPO, etc. . . . NHBD can only be discussed if an unprompted family member brings up organ donation as an important priority of the patient as his/her 'last wish.' If the family discusses the issue prior to a level-of-care decision being made, NHBD will never be considered as an option." This contrasts with another protocol that allows the possibility that families may inquire about organ donation before deciding to withdraw life support and permits OPO personnel to inform them that a decision to withdraw support should not be influenced by any considerations of organ donation. OPO personnel are allowed to return thereafter to discuss donation. About half of the protocols mention the need to inform the family that the patient may not die within the time required to allow donation. In such cases if the patient is in the operating room, he or she will be returned to the intensive care unit (ICU) until expiration.

The amount of information provided to the family during or after informed consent is not clear in many protocols. About half of the protocols describe an informing process. Some are explicit, "The procedures necessary to perfuse and preserve the vascular organs will be explained, as will the necessity for disease testing, tissue typing, and moving to the OR [operating room] in a rapid manner following cardiopulmonary arrest. The family will be told that they may change their decision about donation at any time up to the actual removal of organs. In addition it will be explained that prior to any perfusion of organs, the patient must be declared dead by a physician. If the family so chooses, the OPO Coordinator will again verify consent after the pronouncement of death." Another states that "the OPO Coordinator will sit down with the family and fully explain the NHBD procedure and answer any questions which the family may have."

Some protocols devote little attention to the informing of families, and a few do not mention an explanation of the donation procedure to the family at all. After discussion of donation with the patient or family, many protocols require the OPO coordinator to obtain the necessary written consent. A few others specify the attending physician or attending physician's designee.

OPO AND PROCUREMENT TEAM INTERVENTION BEFORE DEATH

As noted, some OPOs assess donor suitability with various tests (apnea, serology, blood tests, tissue typing, etc.) before decisions to donate are made. The extent of OPO and procurement team preparation of the patient for organ retrieval also differs among protocols and has definite ethical implications. The point at which the procurement team inserts femoral arterial cannulas in anticipation of in situ organ flushing and preservation after death is of particular interest.

Half of the OPO protocols allow the transplant surgeon to insert femoral arterial cannulas before the withdrawal of life support. Ten protocols require consent for cannulation. The other four do not explicitly mention any consent. Eight protocols prescribe cannulation immediately after death is pronounced. The location of withdrawal of life support affects the timing of cannulation in a few protocols. If withdrawal is to take place in the ICU, the transplant physician places cannulas before withdrawal of support with a separate consent from the family. If withdrawal takes place in the OR, cannulas are placed after death. Another protocol implies that the timing of cannulation permits different choices for the location of withdrawal and death. If a cold perfusion catheter is in place, discontinuation of support may take place in the ICU or the OR with family present. If catheters are not in place prior to withdrawal, withdrawal must occur in the OR and family may not be present. The implications are the same. The availability of cannulation and early cooling is compatible with procurement delays caused by transit to the OR and concessions to family presence and sensibilities, or the likelihood of these delays encourages provisions for early cooling.

Yet another protocol seems ambiguous as to when cannulation occurs. This protocol calls for "consent for cannulation of the femoral artery and veins immediately after the declaration of death." In the rest of the protocol's description of procedures, the cannulation step is listed before the termination of support, and statements such as, "the time of death is the start of warm ischemic time on the OPO chart, if cannulae are placed after death" cause further ambiguity. A few protocols are imprecise regarding patient preparation for donation and simply note that the "patient is prepped and draped prior to the withdrawal of support." One protocol allows hospital personnel including the attending physician or the physician pronouncing death to "participate in . . . the procedures to preserve the donor's tissues or organs" if there is a shortage of help.

MEDICATION

The administration of certain medications prior to donor death, in particular the anticoagulant heparin and the vasodilator phentolamine (Regitine), has generated public controversy and led, at least in part, to the request for this report from DHHS. These medications increase blood flow and preserve organs, but some observers allege that they also hasten the death of donors.

OPO NHBD protocols disagree on the procedural use of heparin and phentolamine and the ethics of their use (see Table 5.1).

Of the 29 OPO protocols reviewed, as noted in Table 5.1, 15 specify using heparin or the combination of heparin and phentolamine at some point during the death and donation process. Five OPOs administer heparin prior to termination of life support. One OPO administers heparin at the termination of support before death. Another gives heparin immediately after death is declared and circulates it through the donor's body with chest compression. This is also done in uncontrolled donors by yet another OPO. Two OPOs give heparin and phentolamine before the termination of life support. Single OPOs administer heparin and phentolamine after withdrawal, but before death, or after death but circulated by chest compression (also sometimes as a flush solution). Three OPOs use heparin and phentolamine only after death as part of flush and preservation solutions.

TABLE 5.1. Administration of Heparin and Phentolamine Included in Protocols

No. of OPOs	Medications Administered
5	Heparin before withdrawal of life support
1	Heparin after withdrawal of life support, before declaration of death
2	Heparin after death, circulate with cardiac massage
2	Heparin and phentolamine in intravenous (IV) push before withdrawal of life support
1	Heparin and phentolamine after withdrawal of life support, before declaration of death
1	Heparin and phentolamine after declaration of death, circulate with chest massage
3	Heparin and phentolamine after declaration of death as part of flush solution
15	OPOs that mention using heparin or heparin and phentolamine combination
3	OPOs that explicitly forbid use of heparin and phentolamine or other drugs that "may hasten death"

The remaining 14 OPO protocols either (1) forbid the use of phentolamine and heparin: "This protocol forbids any intervention which intentionally hastens the death of the patient. The administration of medications (such as Regitine and heparin) are *[sic]* forbidden. No interventions are to be justified by their being effective in preserving a more useful transplant or in regulating the time of death"; (2) do not specify the medications to be used—"patient given IV fluids, medications, blood products, etc. to prepare for donation"; or (3) do not mention the use of medications at all, although in some cases it is known that affiliated programs use heparin before support is withdrawn. Other medications used in various protocols include Thorazine, Verapamil, mannitol, cephalosporin, penicillin, insulin, trifluoperazine, and SoluMedrol and other steroids "to reduce ischemic damage."

WITHDRAWAL OF LIFE SUPPORT AND DECLARATION OF DEATH

Withdrawal of life support and declaration of death in controlled NHBDs differ among OPO protocols. In order to avoid conflicts of interest, all protocols explicitly require that the physician who declares death must not be affiliated in any way with the OPO, recovery team, or transplant team. The President's Commission and the Uniform Determination of Death Act define death as the "irreversible cessation of circulatory and respiratory functions." However, each individual physician, under applicable state laws, can determine when cessation is "irreversible," and criteria for the determination of death in NHBDs vary among OPO protocols.

Several protocols thoroughly detail standards for the determination of death by the attending physician or a physician without any conflict of interest: "death shall be pronounced when the patient meets the following cardiopulmonary criteria: 1. confirm correct EKG lead placement, AND 2. confirm a pulse of zero via arterial catheter, AND 3. confirm patient is apneic, AND 4. confirm patient is unresponsive to verbal stimuli, AND 5. A) two minutes of ventricular fibrillation OR B) two minutes of electrical asystole OR C) two minutes of electromechanical disassociation" (capitalization in original). Most protocols refer more vaguely to the determination of death as being performed by the attending physician. Six to eleven (protocol language unclear) protocols specify electronic monitoring of the heart for determination of death after withdrawal of support. Others either use auscultation and palpation to monitor pulse or do not specify methods of determining death.

Twelve OPO protocols dictate that the declaration of death and beginning of organ removal shall occur a few minutes (60 seconds, 2 minutes, 4 to 5 minutes, etc.) after detection of cardiac arrest. Presumably, this window of time is to ensure that the cessation of cardiac and pulmonary function is indeed irreversible. Several protocols declare death and begin procurement immediately "after determination of cardiac arrest," making no reference to any pause after the final heartbeats. It should be remembered that these provisions are for controlled NHBDs.

The variation in timing of the events surrounding death is exemplified by comparing the following protocols. One OPO withdraws support and declares death, continues chest compressions to circulate heparin and phentolamine, and then inserts catheters for cold perfusion before procuring organs. Another OPO performs this sequence in reverse: it inserts cannulas, withdraws support, administers phentolamine and heparin, and then declares death before procuring organs. Still another protocol appears imprecise in its timing of termination of support and declaration of death: "A non-transplant physician is present to pronounce death . . . ventilator is discontinued . . . at the word of the recovery surgeon life support is terminated if not already done . . . at the time of EMD [electronic dissociation], a non-transplant physician will make the declaration of death if not already done."

Most protocols specify an interval during which death must occur following the withdrawal of support if procurement and donation are to continue. This interval averages about 1 hour, with extremes of 30 minutes and 4 hours. A majority of protocols prescribe that in cases where death does not occur within the established time, the family will be notified and patients returned to the ICU until death.

The location of withdrawal of support and the possibility of family attendance are also areas of incongruity. Most protocols allow patient preparation and withdrawal of life support to occur in either the ICU or the OR. A few indicate that the OR has to be scheduled and reserved in advance, before withdrawal of support. Planning ahead for the location of procedures such as withdrawal of life support, determination of death, and initial cooling and procurement seems important given the tight timetable that must be followed to ensure the procurement of viable organs. One protocol views the location of withdrawal of support and patient death as having ethical implications: "To maintain the necessary level of separation between death and donation, life support will be withdrawn in the ICU, CCU [critical care unit], PICU [pediatric ICU], Post-Op, the Emergency Department, or such place, other than the Operating Room, that the patient may be located." In all cases when withdrawal of support followed by declaration of death occurs outside the OR, the patient is promptly transferred to the OR for organ procurement. A few protocols dictate that withdrawal of support is to take place only in the OR in order to "maximize the prospect for survival of transplanted organs."

More than half of the protocols provide some flexibility in location of declaration of death, and many of these mention the family option of attending withdrawal. The remaining protocols either do not mention or do not allow family presence during the withdrawal, death, and donation procedures. Protocols that require withdrawal and death in the OR occasionally state that the family may not be present at this time. A few protocols in which withdrawal and death occur in the ICU explicitly allow families to be at the bedside at this time. The donor is moved to the OR for organ recovery after the family has said its good-byes and left the ICU. Some protocols allow family presence at withdrawal of support and death contingent on the location of these two events. One of these protocols gives the following choice to families: "Protocol A: if discontinuation of life support and death pronouncement *will occur in the OR,* the final viewing of patient by family and friends will occur in the ICU prior to the patient being moved to the OR. The primary care team responsible for discontinuing life support and pronouncement of death will move with the patient or meet the patient in the OR, and retrieval personnel may be present in the OR at the discretion of the attending physician. Protocol B: if discontinuation of life support and death pronouncement will *occur in a private holding area in the OR recovery room,* family may be present, and donor personnel will not enter the patient care area until the family has completed their visitation and death has been pronounced" (emphasis in the original). Another protocol stipulates, "Should a cold perfusion catheter be in place, the terminal wean may take place in the block room of the OR, the isolation room in the recovery room, or the patient's ICU bed. Family members may be present during the terminal wean in either of these locations. If no catheter is in place, the terminal wean shall take place in the OR and no family members may be present."

UNCONTROLLED NHBDs

Several OPOs seem uncertain of the definition of NHBD, especially an uncontrolled donor. Five OPOs represented to the IOM that they do not have an NHBD protocol and do not formally practice recovery and transplantation of organs from NHBDs. Nevertheless, they have occasionally procured organs from patients who arrested in the OR. One OPO representative stated, "My surgeon and I have taken training for pump perfusion for kidneys, and we have recovered organs from heart-beating, brain-dead patients who arrested in the OR. We gave them heparin and cardiac massage until we could get the organs out." These patients—brain-dead donors who arrest unexpectedly before organ procurement—fall into the uncontrolled NHBD category (Maastricht category IV), but in this country such uncontrolled NHBDs often are not formally defined as such by physicians. As noted earlier, they may be considered controlled NHBDs. One physician felt that "everyone in the country practices this type of organ recovery . . . from patients who crash in the OR."

Seven OPOs that said they did not practice procurement of organs from NHBDs have hospitals in their areas that, according to UNOS data, procured organs from NHBDs sometime between 1992 and 1996. Another OPO reported that it has no protocol but has recovered organs from fewer than 10 NHBDs at family request. Still another OPO stated that, although it has no NHBD protocol, hospitals in its area may develop their own. One hospital in this OPO area performs "infrequent NHBD transplants." It seems likely that the NHBDs from this group of OPOs and hospitals include some controlled as well as uncontrolled donors.

Five OPOs have approved protocols explicitly for uncontrolled NHBDs in addition to their controlled NHBD protocols. One of these, however, covers only the salvage of category IV donors whom are resuscitated for a short period to allow organ recovery. The additional issues that arise in uncontrolled donors (primarily categories I and II) include OPO interventions such as cannulation and cooling before family consent is given and decisions about the timing, initiation, and discontinuation of CPR. Because of time restrictions on the viability of organs, cannulation and initial cooling to preserve organs in uncontrolled NHBDs (who have been pronounced dead) is sometimes done without consent if the family is not immediately available. Cooling is intended to keep the option of donation open by allowing the family, once located, a few hours to decide whether or not to give consent to donate organs. One of the four OPO protocols that describe uncontrolled NHBDs allows this type of cannulation and cooling without consent to occur if the family is not immediately present. Two OPOs require that the family be notified of the patient's death and give consent prior to initial core cooling. After consent for cooling, the OPO is contacted and arrives on-site to cannulate and begin perfusion. The remaining uncontrolled NHBD protocols do not specify whether consent for cooling must be obtained; one that covers only category IV does not discuss this issue. Regardless of whether or not cannulation and cooling take place prior to consent, each OPO protocol for uncontrolled NHBDs prohibits actual organ procurement without family consent.

Another procedure sometimes used during uncontrolled NHBD procurement that deserves consideration is the use of CPR after the patient has been pronounced dead. CPR after death is done for the purpose of keeping organs viable by continuing circulation. Drugs such as heparin and phentolamine and others can also be circulated. One protocol states that after determination of death by the attending physician, CPR is resumed in the emergency room (ER) while attempts are made to locate the family. If the family is not located within 30 minutes, CPR is discontinued and organ recovery is not pursued. The protocol that covers category IV donors prescribes CPR and circulation of heparin to allow organ retrieval. One protocol (not uncontrolled) specifically forbids postmortem chest compression.

CONCLUSION

The overall length and detail of OPO protocols for NHBDs vary greatly. Some contain explanations of the donation crisis, the value of NHBDs, the

OPO's philosophy of the donation process, principles, and a detailed protocol. Others are more general, with little reference to important aspects of the process. One protocol is constructed as a framework within which hospitals may tailor their own NHBD protocols. This protocol allows considerable freedom within some areas while setting minimum standards in others. In general, the NHBD protocols received and reviewed by the IOM have been written or approved within the last 4 years. The oldest was revised and approved in 1993, and the most recent was approved in July 1997. With respect to OPOs that have approved protocols in place, it is important to bear in mind that organs are procured from very few NHBDs (only one or two) by most OPOs each year. The fact that there are 25 OPOs with approved NHBD protocols and that UNOS reports 65 NHBDs in 1996 provides confirmation of the low rate of procurement of organs from NHBDs by most OPOs. Currently, OPOs located at hospitals tend to procure more organs from NHBDs.

Review of the NHBD protocols submitted to the IOM reveals a consensus among OPOs in two areas: (1) discussion of organ donation with families and informed consent should take place only after an independent decision to withdraw life support has been made; and (2) the physician who declares death after withdrawal of support shall not be affiliated in any way with the OPO, procurement team, or transplant team. Outside of these two areas, OPO protocols for NHBDs differ greatly. Some variations are merely procedural whereas others imply ethical differences. The criteria for determining death; medical interventions, including the use of heparin and phentolamine, which are directed toward preparation for transplantation rather than donor patient care; intervention by the OPO to assess and prepare the donor before consent for donation and declaration of death; and the timing, approach, and detail of obtaining family consent—all are problematic issues discussed next in this report. A consensus on these issues, expressed in more standardized and detailed protocols would help to avoid conflicts of interest, safeguard quality care for donors and promote procurement of viable organs. The great variation found in OPO protocols and the increasingly urgent demand for more organs suggest the value of a discussion of NHBD programs in the United States with the objective of a more effective use of the costly Organ Procurement and Transplantation Network.

6

Analysis, Findings, and Recommendations

GENERAL PRINCIPLES

The IOM principal investigator, a group of senior special experts, who are not directly involved in transplantation or procurement, and IOM staff met on July 30, 1997, to hear presentations from invited professionals representing medical and surgical transplantation, organ procurement, the bioethics of transplantation, donors, recipients, and the federal government as described in Appendix B. On July 31, an open meeting was held during which the principal investigator and senior special experts discussed issues that they identified as important based on the information provided the previous day, their own experience and expertise, and literature and data made available by the IOM. The analysis, findings, and recommendations reported here were informed, directed, and supported by this discussion. Subsequent reviews and critiques were carried out by the senior special experts and others, including those intimately familiar with all aspects of transplantation as well as donors and recipients.

The project on Non-Heart-Beating Organ Transplantation: Medical and Ethical Issues in Procurement accepted two basic premises at the outset. First, organ transplantation should, as a matter of national policy, be considered a medically necessary part of care for patients with organ failures. It is assumed that the American people will continue to devote resources to this expensive and complex, but life-saving, technology, and it is understood that costs might rise significantly if organ procurement rose to meet demand. The scope of this report does not include a debate on the relative cost-effectiveness of high-technology care. Second, the recovery of organs from NHBDs should be considered a reasonable source of organs whose potential deserves a serious exploration. It was further noted that it would be well to address both controlled and uncontrolled NHBDs. Regardless of current preferences, both of these sources are used today and may be important in the future if supply is to grow. In spite of their cited problems, results of procurement and transplantation of organs from NHBDs apparently can be competitive with those of more ideal donors. It can be concluded, therefore, that the recovery of organs from NHBDs is an important, medically effective and ethically acceptable approach to closing the gap that exists now and will exist in the future between the demand for and the available supply of organs for transplantation.

There is an important message that emerges, in addition, from an extended consideration of the premises, information, and conclusions presented in this report. Organ donation provides an opportunity to restore vital organ function and reduce morbidity and mortality which is of significant societal value. The public, professionals, hospitals, third-party payers, and government should all further the effort to improve levels of organ donation, including more widespread use of donor cards, a greater investment in support of donation, exploration and implementation of more effective procurement methods, enhanced public awareness, and other steps. This effort to provide this value is the context within which policies and procedures of the national transplantation effort are considered, and it is this value, along with the discouraging prospects for major and sufficient increases in donor supply from living and heart-beating donors, that encourages efforts to realize new kinds of donors such as NHBDs.

There are concepts or principles that should be included in the general context. For purposes of the survey described in this report, the IOM, as is common in survey reports, observed individual OPO confidentiality. Nevertheless, the principle should be that OPO policies and protocols are publicly available. Donor families stress that openness and the involvement and approval of interested members of the public are important in protocol development, in OPO governance and transplant program operation, in donor recruitment, and in other public education efforts. Such efforts, carried out through informational material, public advisory groups and boards, and educational campaigns can enhance public trust and support of organ donation and transplantation (Coolican, 1997). Furthermore, because organ donation and transplantation are so closely and intimately related to matters of life and death, meticulous attention should be paid to ethical considerations. Explicit assurance of this attention and a solid ethical foundation for whatever is done in donation and transplantation are the other important elements in public trust and support. This report has identified informed consent, not killing in retrieving organs, respect for donor and family wishes, and prohibition of active euthanasia as among the principles that are important to this ethical foundation. There may also be times when more conservative approaches than those which some might find ethically permissible should be taken in deference to the current state of public perspective and opinion.

Based on discussion among the principal investigator and senior special experts at, and subsequent to the July 31 meeting, it was concluded that five headings encompassed the problems and issues that might fruitfully be investigated and, insofar as possible, resolved. These are: (1) policies and oversight, (2) medical interventions and ethics, (3) conflicts of interest, (4) determination of death, and (5) families. Because the request for this study explicitly required a focus on donors, organ procurement and retrieval, they did not include any recipient issues.

POLICIES AND OVERSIGHT

Specific and important pressures are brought to bear during procurement and preparation for transplantation of organs from NHBDs, both controlled and uncontrolled, that exceed those on other types of donors. These pressures generate greater risks of premature cessation of treatment or nonbeneficial or lifeshortening interventions in a living patient, conflicts of interest between care and donation and premature declaration of death, among others. Therefore, policies for all categories of NHBDs must be different from policies for brain-dead (heart-beating) and living donors, although as Robertson (1993) has pointed out, it is not clear that the ethics differ materially among them.

A survey of the NHBD policies and protocols of all active OPOs has been described in detail in chapter 5. This survey revealed importantly that 34 of 63 OPOs had NHBD protocols approved (25) or in differing stages of development (9). As a reflection perhaps of the historical level of local autonomy of OPOs, and perhaps not surprisingly, there was substantial variation among protocols in principles cited and scope and detail of coverage. There were important and sometimes contradictory differences in ethically problematic provisions such as those regarding the timing and kinds of organ-conserving interventions and the standards for determining death. Five OPOs had protocols covering uncontrolled as well as controlled NHBDs, and some OPOs were recovering organs from one or the other kind of NHBD without protocols. The protocols were uniform in separating discussions and decisions on withdrawal of life support from those on donation and in requiring the independence of those responsible for declaration of death from those involved in procurement.

The fact that OPO NHBD protocols differ is not by itself necessarily a problem. Accepted geographic variation in medical practice, local custom, differences in demographic and social characteristics, and the need to accommodate the circumstances of OPOs that cover greatly varying population sizes and numbers of hospitals or transplant centers should be taken into account in protocol content. Protocols also should be able to respond to changes in practice, advances in technology, evolving public views in matters such as withdrawal of life support, or new laws at various jurisdictional levels such as those presuming consent for, or otherwise authorizing cannulation and cooling. The myriad individual circumstances of patients and the differences in hospitals' and programs' geography, size, capacity, numbers, and types of personnel, as well as their experience and expertise, argue for flexibility in protocols and a commitment to live up to the spirit of a sound, ethical policy rather than an attempt to predict every possible contingency.

On the other hand, protocols should not be inconsistent among OPOs and hospitals in ways that raise questions about the motives and priorities of transplant programs or the scientific and ethical standards of care for donor patients. Fundamental scientific and ethical principles do not vary from region to region. Some of the current anomalies could be damaging to public confidence and in this way destructive to the crucial, life-saving organ donation effort. Organ transplantation is a nationwide effort, and there should be some coherence and uniformity across the country. Among the national initiatives are programs for data collection, organ allocation, OPO certification and oversight from the Health Care Financing Administration (HCFA), oversight from the Health Resources and Services Administration (HRSA), and significant federal funding. Smaller local efforts may benefit from access to the ethical or other expertise available on a national basis. New entrants to transplantation and procurement may find reassurance if there are some national guidelines. A sense that an agreed on, consistent community standard is being met may help these programs to design and be comfortable with their own protocols and policies. A local program that creates adverse public reaction may come to national notice and prejudice the entire national effort.

The European transplant community's 12 Maastricht Statements and Recommendations require (No. 5) that "no NHBD program should be started without a written protocol approved by the local medical ethical committee" (Kootstra, 1995). The Maastricht Statements and Recommendations also list performance and procedural requirements that transplant programs should observe. In a similar fashion, the key principles and provisions in this report can justifiably form a consistent part of NHBD transplantation in all regions of the United States with room left to accommodate other content that provides the necessary flexibility noted above. Such principles and provisions should be nationally required; this could involve consultation, review, and acceptance from those involved in transplantation, which includes donors, recipients, and the public.

Procurement of organs from any kind of NHBD takes hospitals and procurement organizations into difficult ethical and medical territory, exposing them to risks of error or controversial practices and resulting public disapproval. The policies and procedures to be followed should be thought through in advance and codified in a written protocol. Ways should be found to bring health care, ethics, and public representation, particularly organ donors, donor families, and transplant patients, into the process of developing and approving such a protocol. All protocols should define and describe the kinds and characteristics of donors from whom organs will be procured under the protocol. Because the deadly and growing gap between donor supply and demand will not be closed without new sources of organs, procurement organizations should consider covering all categories of uncontrolled as well as controlled NHBDs under their protocols. They also should decide whether or not to cover conscious donors who can give consent as well as unconscious donors whose families or surrogates consent. The risks and procedures will differ significantly among the various categories of donors. For example, conscious donors who can give consent present particular problems in weaning from life-sustaining treatment, almost always artificial ventilation, without inappropriate hastening of death by pain control and sedation, even though there is essentially 100% confidence that death is inevitable shortly in such patients, and all ethical and family considerations are already satisfactorily in place. Uncontrolled NHBDs such as those in categories I or II, who could not be resuscitated after a heart attack, present the danger that prematurely abandoning resuscitation to turn to organ donation may forfeit the life of a patient who is otherwise a salvageable, competent person. The issues of timing and determination of death do not arise in category IV uncontrolled NHBDs because the patient has already been determined (brain) dead.

Under the headings that follow the IOM recommends certain principles and provisions that should be included in all protocols. This report does not cover all desirable content. The IOM focused on issues that were relevant to the charge of the sponsors of this project, that appeared to need attention at present, and that could be addressed with the time and resources available. Appropriate, additional provisions have been included in many protocols that reflect local considerations. These include ruling in or out various classes of patients by diagnosis, physical or mental condition, or other factors, specific responsibilities of various personnel, and other particular safeguards with respect to conflicts of interest between donor patient care and donation, including ethical consultation and the role of ethics committees, special arbiters, timing of various steps, and the like.

Certain context and principles for protocols have already been noted, such as the social value of donation, disclosure and openness, and the emphasis on a solid ethical basis for protocol provisions. The principles that donation not cause the death of donors and that there be no interventions that might constitute active euthanasia must be inviolate. These principles, respect for donor and family wishes, the primacy of consent based on disclosure and a commitment to informing, and allowing consent to be withdrawn at any time up to the beginning of organ removal are also an important context within which protocols should be developed.

This report concludes under this first heading that a written protocol that is completely open and available to the public should be a requirement for the procurement and transplantation of organs from NHBDs. Protocols should have some minimal content and uniformity of coverage, content, principles, and definitions as part of a nationwide NHBD effort and as indicated in this report. As the medical, procedural, and ethical concerns about NHBDs are addressed in this report and elsewhere and to the extent that they are resolved, little is gained if the progress made is not reflected in policy and behavior when and where NHBD transplantation is taking place. The issues identified in this report and, in fact, the important progress already made in identifying problems and best practice and in addressing central medical and ethical questions are important elements for a high standard of care in transplantation and for generating both public confidence in the process of donation and public willingness to volunteer. Little purpose is served if these elements exist in a vacuum.

MEDICAL INTERVENTIONS AND ETHICS

A number of important concerns have been identified under the second heading, **medical interventions and ethics.** First, this report concludes that it is essential to acknowledge that there must and should be interventions undertaken in the management of a patient for whom consent to become an organ donor has been given, including heart-beating or non-heart-beating, that would not be undertaken in a nondonor patient with similar medical condition. These interventions are taken in furtherance of a donation process that is effective and that safeguards the patient. Some are more common in heart-beating donors (Scheinkestel et al., 1995). Others might be accepted treatment of non-donor patients. This includes those that resuscitate or sustain life and maintain organ function, but under the circumstances of an actual donor patient, perhaps because of the severity of the damage due to injury or disease or because of a prior decision to forgo further treatment, their administration or the timing of their administration raises questions of whose welfare is being served. Still other interventions include organ conservation measures by specific preservation and treatment technologies or by monitoring, which can also ensure that life has ended and organ removal is not premature.

These matters can be described in more detail as those that critically involve (1) timing of interventions; (2) characterization of interventions—those that are provided to conserve organs to be donated also positively affect donor patient medical status, and may or may not prolong dying in the process; those that conserve organs to be donated and do no harm to the donor patient; those that conserve organs and are potentially harmful to the donor patient, and those that are invasive and/or definitely harmful; and (3) family and surrogate informed consent.

Interventions can also be examined as to whether they involve (1) resuscitation, performed primarily for the purpose of enabling a patient to become a donor; (2) monitoring, such as arterial and urethral catheters, to support and inform donation care rather than patient care; (3) insertion and use of perfusion cannulas for organ preservation and, potentially, for organ viability screening; (4) patient stabilization measures, especially in severely brain-damaged patients, such as heating or cooling blankets for temperature control, transfusions and other IV fluids, antibiotics, and hormones or other pharmaceuticals for control of vital functions when aggressive means would ordinarily be forgone; and (5) organ-protecting agents such as anticoagulants, vasodilators, diuretics (osmotic), steroids, and other more experimental agents to inhibit the formation of or to scavenge free radicals (allopurinol, superoxide dismutase), control prostaglandin activity, and the like (D'Alessandro et al., 1995b; Hoshino et al., 1988). Many of the latter agents will likely be limited to postmortem organ perfusion.

As noted, some of these interventions might be accepted treatment of severely ill patients, but they are used here in the context of the NHBD in the sense that they must either by their nature be directed primarily or exclusively at the organs to be transplanted or in the circumstances of a severely ill patient be of questionable use or timing when the usual course might be to avoid aggressive treatment and to let the patient die. Although it referred to potential heart-beating, rather than non-heart-beating, donors, a recent financial review (Grossman et al., 1996) provided a quantitative example of the extent to which designation as a donor generates a change in care that can then no longer be assigned to the welfare of the patient but is directed toward organ procurement. Of the average $33,997 hospital stay cost, $17,385 was considered "futile" for the patient, but probably "necessary for improved organ procurement rates." With the understanding that designation as a donor undoubtedly changes, in a similar way, what happens to a NHBD patient, the overarching questions here include the following: is this change and are these interventions ethically acceptable; is the timing of these interventions ethically problematic; for which interventions is informed consent a requirement; and are there modifying conditions to the use of these interventions that might be necessary or helpful?

Within the context of the social value of enhancing donation and the other principles and provisions previously noted, this report concludes that these interventions can be appropriate, although only two are discussed in detail. They should be thought through in advance and be part of the approved protocol. There may be need for some flexibility since not every possible circumstance can be predicted, but provision should be made to err in the direction of disclosure, informing, and obtaining consent. Whatever the level of detail, donor families should, at a minimum, understand that to ensure the best results, some actions will be taken that are specific to the donation process and not of benefit to donor patient care. However, informed consent by itself does not allow or excuse interventions that are injurious or actively life-shortening.

The IOM focused on two interventions, administration of anticoagulants and vasodilators (e.g., heparin and phentolamine) and arterial cannulation for cooling, that are particularly relevant to the reasons for this report. Some have asked whether the principle of double effect might not be germane to the issues involved in interventions such as the administration of heparin and phentolamine. That is, the intentional achievement of a good effect, procurement of a lifesaving organ from a donor, permits the risk and possible occurrence of an unintended bad effect, hastening the death of the donor. Experts have argued that this principle may be applicable in some donor or transplantation situations (Childress, 1993). It is very unlikely that heparin and phentolamine would be part of nondonor patient care in medical circumstances similar to those of NHBDs. In certain patients under certain circumstances, these drugs may actively hasten death although no specific instance of this in any donor has been reported. While withdrawal of life support obviously, and ethically, hastens death in NHBDs, it is not an active lethal intervention taken to benefit mostly unknown and unrelated other individuals. This is a heavy potential burden for the principle of double effect, and there is no consensus about whether the principle can bear it.

In the occasional NHBD with ongoing intracranial bleeding or deficiencies in blood volume, the administration of anticoagulants or vasodilators such as heparin or phentolamine is not indicated because it could actively cause death. On the other hand, the administration of these drugs through circulation by chest compression or in a flush solution after death does not harm the donor and is justifiable as routine. Heparin and phentolamine, however, are recommended frequently during the donation process, based on clinical experience and scientific evidence that they enhance donor organ quality and graft results and usually can be safely used (D'Alessandro, 1997; Miller et al., 1974). Although prescription of these drugs during organ procurement is deemed useful and is undoubtedly safe in the majority of instances (Gould et al., 1980), a blanket policy cannot be recommended because of possible untoward effects in some donor patients.

Physicians responsible for the care of individual donors should be able to make a clinical judgment on the advisability of using either heparin or phentolamine or both without hastening donor death. This report recommends that individual clinical judgments be made and also that consideration be given to involving the donor's attending physician as either the responsible prescriber or a required consultant or co-decision maker with the procurement or transplant team to improve patient protection, lessen conflicts of interest, and strengthen public confidence. Protocols should note that donor families should be specifically informed on these matters, or more generally advised and given an opportunity to question further, that certain interventions (and the determination of death) may involve their own attending physicians on a case-by-case basis to safeguard patient interests. Provisions for informed consent for heparin and requiring that the order for heparin originate with the attending physician are found in existing NHBD protocols, albeit very rarely.

Review of cases by a relevant committee of the involved facility is a final safeguard which may be desirable. Actions such as whether the attending physician or his designee signed or cosigned an order for an intervention (e.g., phentolamine) or whether chart notes indicate compliance with standards and procedures (e.g., those used in the determination of death) are susceptible to review and control at a subsequent time. Ethics committees would be appropriate for this, although a recent report sheds some doubt on their readiness for this task (Spielman and Verhulst, 1997).

Cannulas can be inserted through leg arteries and veins into major abdominal arteries and veins to allow postmortem organ cooling and preservation by perfusion through the blood vessels of internal donor organs with special cold solutions. Many programs believe that rapid organ flushing and cooling, also associated with general cooling through infusion of cold solutions into the abdominal cavity, are important in recovering viable organs from NHBDs, organs that have not suffered the accelerated deterioration that accompanies loss of circulation in an uncooled body. In controlled NHBDs, decisions to withdraw life-sustaining measures are followed by decisions to donate. Thereafter, decisions can be made to cannulate before the withdrawal of life support, with the intent to perfuse as soon as cardiopulmonary death has been pronounced. Cannulation can also be performed later in the course of events, including immediately after death. Perfusion, since it usually involves solutions that will stop heart action immediately, must always await the declaration of death. Cannulation does not hasten death, and it is important in preparing for rapid initiation of organ preservation and enhancing the chances of obtaining quality donor organs and the best graft results for recipients. Cannulation is invasive, and, in a conscious person, painful. The report finds that cannulation is acceptable in controlled NHBDs after a decision to donate is made and beginning just before withdrawal of life support or at any time thereafter, but it recommends that consent always be explicitly required and that local anesthesia be used if needed. The issue of cannulation can be resolved at the time consent for organ donation is discussed.

With the possible exception of category IV uncontrolled NHBDs, where donation (and even cannulation) may have been discussed, the great majority of uncontrolled NHBDs suffer cardiopulmonary death unexpectedly and most often without family decisionmakers immediately at hand to give consent for measures such as cannulation and cooling. At the same time, the pressure for cooling is greatest in these donors because they are likely to have the longest intervals of organs unrecovered in the body at normal body temperature. These organs suffer the greatest deterioration, have the most frequent delayed function, and offer lower chances of long-term graft survival. As noted earlier, a delay of

30 or 45 minutes, which many European programs accept, may result in as high as 100% delayed kidney function and has so far ruled out transplantation of other organs (D'Alessandro et al., 1995b; Kootstra and Daemen, 1995). This has led to laws that allow cooling without consent in other countries and in three jurisdictions in the United States and to the practice of nonconsensual cooling, without statutory authority, in Illinois (UNOS, 1992), which was subsequently abandoned. The importance of cooling and preservation to the viability and function of NHBD organs, especially in uncontrolled NHBD cases; the likelihood that actual mechanical perfusion and cooling are superior to cooling alone (Southard and Belzer, 1995; Light et al., 1994); and the possibility that perfusion characteristics may allow useful screening for organ viability (Daemen et al., 1997) make the questions of timing, disclosure, and consent involving insertion of cannulas and initiation of cooling particularly prominent.

After a determination that further resuscitation efforts are futile and a declaration of cardiopulmonary death, the insertion of cannulas and the initiation of cooling pending location of family decision makers and receipt of consent for donation are problematic but can be considered. Patients with valid organ donor cards or other advance directives that grant permission are patients with legal consent, and this report concludes that in such instances, cannulation, cooling, and organ retrieval should proceed consistent with the donor patient's clear wishes. Individual procurement organizations or programs generally discontinue organ preservation and recovery if families are located and object, given the possibility of adverse public reaction. Ignoring the expressed wishes of the true donor in such a way is considered pragmatic local policy, but it is not a legal necessity, and it is hard to imagine how nonadherence to legal advance directives could be justified as a national policy statement.

In cases without donor cards or family consent, procurement organizations and transplant programs face decisions involving ethical concerns that are not definitely resolved. On the one hand, there is a prevailing sense that the public is likely to disapprove of nonconsensual cannulation and cooling. Specific, strong opposition was expressed in surveys in three cities (Arnold, 1997), and public concerns, noted earlier from other surveys, about inadequate treatment efforts on behalf of donors or premature initiation of donation may reflect similar sentiments. It is noteworthy that in Florida a law that presumes consent for cooling goes unimplemented by transplant programs unwilling to test public opinion. Serious damage to donation efforts could be done if unauthorized cannulation generated significant public discontent. Finally, modifiers such as "minimally" do not change the fact that cannulation and cooling constitute an invasive procedure that may be very objectionable or if enough people find this offensive (and the numbers are not known), it might come to be considered definitely unethical without consent. It might also provoke feelings strong enough to generate a search for legal remedies for mutilation of the corpse, among others.

On the other hand, many people approve. As noted, there are laws in three major U.S. jurisdictions and a number of developed Western democracies that allow cannulation without consent. Many strongly believe in the social value of strengthening organ donation. More and better organs through better and earlier preservation are among the ways to realize that value. Organs that are in good condition may spare recipients the increased likelihood of the pain, morbidity, depression, and death associated with marginal grafts that have higher failure rates. It is argued, and evidence and testimonials have been presented (Coolican, 1997—see Appendix B; Douglass and Daly, 1995), that families take comfort and meaning from the knowledge that their loved one's organs live on and sustain life in other human beings. Organ donation can snatch a small victory from the pain of unexpected death. On a practical level, nonconsensual cannulation has been carried out a number of times and continues to be practiced, it is said, from time to time in the United States without generating any major controversy. This does not seem a strong argument in its favor, however.

Perhaps further study and discussion should be pursued. A consensus on the ethics might be reached, and public opinion may evolve or be favorably influenced through continued education and information. Time may, therefore, provide an answer. Local procurement organizations and programs are certainly free to practice nonconsensual cooling in jurisdictions with statutory authority or to consider it in other parts of the country. Nevertheless, there are risks to proceeding without consent, and offended families are unlikely to be pacified by any of the justifications listed in this report. Cannulation and cooling without consent may be a situation in which a decision based on deference to what the public is prepared to accept may be the wisest policy at the moment.

CONFLICTS OF INTEREST

The third heading, **conflicts of interest**, has generated the most consistent approaches in protocols reviewed by the IOM. All procurement organizations and transplant programs appear to understand the need for strong safeguards to ensure that conflicts of interest do not lead to violations of prevailing medical and ethical standards of care for patients who may become or already are designated donors. These safeguards require separating major decisions and discussions in patient care (withdrawal of life support, discontinuing CPR, and declaration of death) from major decisions and discussions in organ donation and transplantation (obtaining consent for donation and other transplant-related procedures and involvement in the actual process of organ retrieval). Such safeguards include scrupulous separation of patient care personnel from procurement and transplant personnel. In some cases, such as determination of death, this separation is pursuant to law (Martin, 1970). They include spacing in time, as distinct events, discussions concerning withdrawal of support and discussions about consent to donation. They also include assigning responsibility for the declaration of death and important aspects of medical management during the dying and donation process, such as weaning from life support, resuscitation decisions, and perhaps in some ways decisions on organ-conserving interventions that may be harmful in certain patients under certain conditions, to attending physicians who are responsible for patient care and not to the physicians who are responsible for organ procurement and transplantation. The decisions made and the care delivered at the time of withdrawal of life-sustaining treatment in the case of controlled NHBDs or at the time of CPR in uncontrolled NHBDs pose particularly challenging conflicts of interest. In the former instance, interventions intended to ensure comfort and pain relief may also be those that can hasten death. In the latter instance, the proper time to discontinue CPR may be subjective and dependent on an assessment of the circumstances of the individual case. Given the importance of the timing of events to organ viability, the types and timing of interventions or decisions on CPR may be perceived to have been influenced by the demands of transplantation. The pressures for a prompt and predictable declaration of death and the complete dependence of patients at these critical times require particular attention to conflict of interest issues and safeguards. As a practical matter, resident physicians may well be those closest to patients and families and therefore most suited to assume some roles in donor care and transplantation. Provision for their involvement under supervision may be desirable.

By agreement with hospitals or under state law OPOs are becoming involved through routine referral and mandatory notification about dying patients. As a result, they are being introduced, and the subject of donation is being introduced from time to time at earlier stages in the course of care of terminal patients when separation of life support withdrawal decisions from the possibility of donation is important. This report is not recommending specific new safeguards to handle the conflicts of interest between withdrawal and donation. Nevertheless, the changes in procedure that follow more aggressive and successful procurement increase the potential for these conflicts. Early interventions are reviewed in chapter 5 of this report and suggest that further thought on the implications of earlier and more pervasive approaches may be needed.

Finally, some NHBD patients may receive care at nontransplant facilities, after which their organs are sent to transplant centers. There are many more hospitals that provide donors (1,300) than there are transplant centers (275). Nevertheless, many NHBD patients are managed at transplant centers. Here, personnel, even if not part of the transplant program, are likely to be at least aware of the possible benefits in prestige, research support, patient care reimbursement, and staff recruitment that may accompany a successful, growing transplant program. Such an "institutional bias" toward improving the supply of donor organs may be difficult to completely resolve by any conflict of interest safeguards (Frader, 1993). Disclosure to donor families that in such facilities procurement efforts may be more intense and the needs of a transplant program will be in the staff's minds seems a reasonable measure for recognizing and managing this possible bias.

A prevailing attitude in favor of searching out and procuring donors may encourage extra steps to support and maintain patients whose condition suggests that they could go on to become possible donors if life can be sustained. This kind of admixture of patient care and donation objectives provides sustaining care interventions for patients, meets obligations to enhance organ donation, and is reasonable as long as patient and family needs are met within a policy of openness. It is difficult or impossible even to isolate the donation effort in such instances. More overt and less directly patient-supportive steps are not acceptable before donation has been discussed with families and consent given. This report finds that conflict of interest safeguards are among the most important aspects of protocols. Many conflicts of interest provisions were identified in chapter 5, and the particular provision discussed in this chapter should be part of NHBD protocols. Requiring non-heart-beating donation to be initiated always by the family and never at the suggestion of patient care or procurement staff, as provided in one existing protocol, is a level of strictness that this report finds is a local option, not a necessity. Complete elimination of conflicts and separation of withdrawal and donation are probably impossible. Removing hospital or procurement staff from the request process does not ensure completely disinterested family decision making, or preclude the improper influence of institutional or other considerations on the acceptance of donation by professional staff. Therefore it is not recommended.

DETERMINATION OF DEATH

This report has addressed two important concerns under the fourth heading, **determination of death**. The definition of cardiopulmonary death as "irreversible cessation of circulatory and respiratory functions" is short and simple. The current variability and, arguably, confusion in practices for the determination of donor death as reflected in existing protocols for controlled NHBDs arise from the controversy over what constitutes "irreversible" and because great precision in the moment of death is rarely crucial in general practice, from the custom of using simple and imprecise standards and technologies to determine death. A little more time can make the diagnosis obvious but, in donors, may result in organs of poor or unusable quality. Timing of death is crucial in NHBD organ procurement, however. Because the incentives are toward the earliest possible determination, NHBD policies that do not have a clear definition with a credible mechanism and standards leave procurement organizations and transplant programs open to charges of inadequate safeguards and practices for preventing premature determination of death and removal of organs.

Some protocols offer very little detail regarding the determination of death. Some controlled NHBD policies specify cessation of circulatory function measured in the usual way but supported by absence of electrocardiographic evidence of heartbeat (no meaningful electrical activity, ventricular fibrillation, or electromechanical dissociation) for 2 minutes. Other programs, particularly in Europe and particularly for uncontrolled NHBDs, specify 10 minutes of cessation measured in various ways. Still another option provides more local discretion: "Irreversibility of cardiopulmonary function is recognized by persistent cessation during an appropriate period of observation and/or trial of therapy. In clinical situations where death is expected, where the cause has been gradual and where irregular, agonal respirations, or cardiac activity finally ceases, the period of observation following the cessation of cardiopulmonary function may need to be only a few minutes in order to establish death. When a possible death is unobserved, unexpected, or sudden, the examination may need to be more detailed or extend over a longer period while appropriate resuscitative efforts are maintained as a test for cardiovascular responsiveness" (U.S. organ procurement and transplant program NHBD policy).

There is an important need for clear definition, method, and standards for determination of death. This involves questions of which and how many physicians should be involved, tests used, the timing, and the consideration given to individual circumstances or kinds of patients that might modify the approach. The key concern is not whether circulation and respiration have ceased, but whether they have irreversibly done so.

Attempts to clarify the meaning of irreversible have revolved around a number of questions. Withdrawal of life support undoubtedly leads to cessation of circulatory function that, even if the possibility of spontaneous return of effective heartbeat is left aside, might sometimes be reversed if life support were restored or other resuscitative measures were initiated. In the situation of the controlled NHBD, however, a valid refusal of further treatment is in hand, and a decision has been made to withdraw life support with an understanding of the consequences. At some interval after the last heartbeat because in this instance medical intervention is not to be attempted, the heart will not have the capacity to autoresuscitate and circulatory failure will be irreversible. Unfortunately, no scientific studies allow a definite conclusion on how long this interval might be. Protocols and practices in the United States and other countries vary significantly in defining this interval, which reflects the lack of scientific certainty. As noted in chapter 5, some controlled NHBD protocols take into account the manner of death, allowing a shorter interval after a longer agonal period. Some do not require any elapsed time, and some leave the definition to the attending physician's discretion. Others prescribe intervals of 1, 2, or 5 minutes or yet other timing. Much longer time periods are accepted in uncontrolled NHBDs, up to 1 hour, with consequences that have been described in other chapters of this report. The shorter intervals between cessation of circulation and determination of death are problematic as to the assurance of irreversibility. Intervals such as 2 minutes are not supported by any experimental data on the probability of autoresuscitation and are too short to support a determination of brain death due to circulatory arrest (Lynn, 1993). On the other hand, recent enactment by the Swiss National Academy of Medical Sciences of official guidelines on cardiac death, with respect to potential organ donation for uncontrolled NHBDs, that specify 30 minutes of unsuccessful cardiopulmonary resuscitation under hospital conditions has raised a number of issues. Among these is the advisability of a definition of death that is defined specifically in terms of organ donation and that has caused the availability of NHBDs to decrease by 50% (Schlumpf et al., 1997).

Clarification of the meaning of irreversibility and of the determination of death must rest on expert medical opinion. The fact that the controlled NHBD is a severely ill or injured patient, with impaired physiology and near death, informs this opinion. This is the context in which the value of enhancing donation and procuring organs in a timely way is weighed against the ability of organs to tolerate short periods of circulatory failure and the requirement that the public be given credible and meaningful assurance that donor care has not been compromised, and that donors have died and organs are not prematurely being removed. In the final analysis, however, the opinion must and indeed does rest on expert judgment that the interval is long enough to ensure that the probability of return of circulatory function is vanishingly small. In addition, although this is not relevant to a determination of death, the interval of absent circulation recommended here will, in a donor with normal body temperature, produce irreversible brain damage.* In patients with depressed body temperatures, death is more difficult to determine; time and resource constraints did not allow a thorough exploration of this challenging situation in this report, however. Based on expert information and advice from its senior special experts, this report recommends that in controlled NHBDs, an interval of at least 5 minutes elapse after complete cessation of circulatory function, as measured by standards described later in this chapter, before death is pronounced and organ perfusion or removal begins. It should be noted that the insertion of cannulas, if they are not already in place, can be carried out during the 5-minute wait after the heart stops. Uniform adoption of this recommendation which is on the conservative end of the current range, could ensure that death has occurred, diminish the appearance of haste and reassure the public, and eliminate the uncomfortable situation whereby a donor could be defined as dead in one OPO region and still, however briefly, be defined as alive in another. Since, in the final analysis, this recommendation is only an expert judgment, data should be collected to validate an interval. Clearly, if a 5-minute interval is widely used, within a short time a large number of observations on reversibility during a less than 5-minute interval could be

---

*"Normothermic no-flow of 5 to 20 min reversed by standard [resuscitation] or CPR, however, is still followed by various degrees of permanent multifocal brain damage" (Safar, 1997, p. 560).

collected. These observations might be helpful in confirming a 5-minute interval or providing evidence to change from 5 minutes to a shorter interval based on actual clinical data.

Uncontrolled NHBDs present a different set of concerns. Category IV uncontrolled donors are already dead by neurologic criteria. Although they have suffered unexpected cardiac arrest, they are like heart-beating donors who do not pose questions of definition or determination of cardiopulmonary death because death has already been pronounced. CPR and other life support are relevant to organ preservation in these donors, not to a determination of death, and no interval of arrest is at issue. CPR is involved in other uncontrolled NHBDs who suffer unexpected cardiopulmonary arrest yet may have considerable potential for a return to normal life. In these donors there are major concerns regarding the vigor and duration of attempts to restore circulation, the standards for determining death, and the timing of organ removal.

Uncontrolled NHBDs are a trivial percentage of donors currently, but in theory they could comprise the largest group. Less than 10% of OPOs have protocols covering uncontrolled NHBDs, and few express an interest in expanding efforts in this direction. Nevertheless, the potential of this group, the rather ad hoc current approach, and the procurement of some of these donors scattered among OPOs, often without protocols, suggest that relevant issues should be explored and resolved to the extent possible. The interests of the uncontrolled donor patient in a lengthy and intense effort to restore circulation and the interests of the patients who await organ procurement and transplantation in a brief effort and a short interval of arrest that leaves donor organs in the best condition are in powerful potential conflict. Most CPR is not successful, but long-term return of cardiopulmonary function and return to normal life after several hours of CPR are not unheard of. The circumstantial events and medical status of those who suffer unexpected cardiopulmonary arrest are enormously varied. It is difficult, therefore, to design a uniform approach to the determination of death in uncontrolled NHBDs. The approach of the Swiss Academy of Medical Sciences requiring 30 minutes minimum duration of hospital CPR has been mentioned earlier, and major European programs have recommended a general rule of 10 minutes of absent heartbeat after termination of resuscitative efforts before perfusion or organ retrieval (Kootstra and Daemen, 1995).

Continued evaluation and discussion of the determination of death in uncontrolled NHBDs are recommended. In the meantime, given the great individuality of these donors' circumstances, the individual physicians responsible for caring for them should make decisions on duration of CPR and the interval of absent function necessary to determine death based on their best medical judgment under the particular conditions of each situation. Care of these patients must be completely independent of any consideration of organ donation. The societal value of enhancing organ donation should encourage requests to families of potential uncontrolled NHBDs. The necessity for separation of care from organ procurement and the tight time limits required by medical events, however, may make successful donation difficult unless there is a donor card or until some resolution of the issues discussed earlier with respect to cannulation and cooling allows early cooling and more time to properly carry out the steps necessary for arranging donation. Continued discussion, research, and experience, along with local decision making, could in the interim indicate directions for the future.

A review of current NHBD protocols does not provide a sense that there is a prevailing understanding of the "accepted medical standards" mentioned in law by which cardiopulmonary death is to be determined. As described earlier, protocols vary from no specifics on determination, to the use of palpation and auscultation, to electronic monitoring, to specific descriptions of electrocardiographic results and other confirmatory tests. For the definition of death recommended in this report for controlled NHBDs—or any definition that includes a specific time interval of absent heart function—to be meaningful, an unambiguous time of cessation of function and monitoring to detect any return of function is required. This report recommends, in adhering to the controlled NHBD definition of at least 5 minutes of absent heart function, that accepted medical detection standards include electrocardiographic changes consistent with absent heart function by electronic monitoring and zero pulse pressure as determined by monitoring through an arterial catheter. These standards would require proper placement of electrocardiographic leads and monitoring of cardiac electric activity and the placement of an arterial line (cooling cannulas or a monitoring catheter, which would often be in place anyway) and monitoring of blood pressure. Other findings clearly will also be present, such as absence of breathing and unresponsiveness to stimuli, and notation of these in protocols at local option could be useful.

FAMILIES

This report has explored a number of organizational, procedural, and medical issues important to the national transplantation effort. A nontechnical fifth heading—**families**—is included to reflect the primacy of the principle of respect for donor and donor family wishes and to provide a reminder and some recommendations regarding the essential role of families. Living donors and those heart-beating and non-heart-beating donors who have executed a valid donor card or other advance directive are, as individual members of the public, essential to transplantation. The support of donor families is just as essential. Without them the national effort would amount to a fraction of its present size and hope for future increases in supply would be dim indeed. Procurement organizations and transplant programs undoubtedly recognize that attention to and involvement of families is compassionate, quality medical practice and, in a practical sense, crucial to maintenance and improvement of a national donor effort. By no means do all protocols reflect this, however, although what donor families want and deserve is clear (National Kidney Foundation, 1994).

The focus here is on a number of issues that could be included in protocols. Protocols require that discussions of donor care, withdrawal of treatment, and determination of death be separated from discussions of donation for reasons of conflict of interest. Also, requests for consent are more likely to be successful if these discussions are decoupled, as noted earlier. This separation is important to donor families, and procedures should be designed to properly accommodate this reason as much as the others. Families need time to understand the medical situation and come to terms with their personal tragedy. They also appreciate and benefit from privacy during these times. The circumstances and the separation of discussions should respond to this need.

Results of several surveys included in this report indicate that families often do not understand the meaning of brain death and feel that they needed, but did not receive, more information and explanation of this and other matters related to the care and potential of the patient for donation. The Bill of Rights for Donor Families emphasizes the needs for information, explanation, and the opportunity to understand, with a properly prepared and trained person, the details of a prospective donor's situation and the implications for the family. The value of follow-up is an issue related to this. Many donor families want information on what organs were removed, how they were used, and the results in transplant recipients. This report takes no position on interactions between donor families and recipients and their families. Many families would also appreciate some follow-up support of the kind mentioned in the Bill of Rights for Donor Families. It is to be hoped that attending physicians and responsible resident physicians would continue to have an interest in donor families and be willing to discuss and explain matters to them, to visit on occasion, and to be willing to help with follow-up questions.

Families are customarily afforded considerable latitude to be with patients who are not donors while they are critically ill and dying. The fact of donation should limit as little as possible, preferably not at all, the opportunities for families to attend patients in the same way they would if organ donation was not contemplated. It is recommended that hospitals arrange for some non-OR site where families can be with patients until death, if this is their wish. If this is not their wish the advantages of an OR site may dictate that setting for withdrawal. Individual facilities have different physical layouts and differing potential for accommodating families, so individual solutions will vary. Procurement organizations and transplant programs should review their protocols and procedures to consider whether there has been adequate consideration of donor family needs to attend patients. Families who will be in attendance (indeed all families) should also be fully informed of the possibilities that death may not occur soon enough to permit donation and that, in dying, an occasional respiratory effort or electrical response on cardiogram does not represent return of function.

Finally, procurement organizations, transplant facilities, and government and other payers should review experience and payment rules to determine if donor families are at risk for any expenses that are part of the donation process or that because they are not part of routine patient care, are incurred in anticipation of, and are the responsibility of, the donor process whether it occurs or not. Donor families should not be penalized for altruistically contributing to the social good by enhancing organ procurement and for consenting to make a contribution to the national transplantation program. Several NHBD protocols reviewed in this report already provide that no costs after consent for donation will be borne by donor families whether or not donation is successfully accomplished.

This report has reviewed the history of solid organ transplantation and the current balance between supply and demand. Pursuant to an investigation of the current usage and results of organ recovery from NHBDs, it is concluded that controlled and uncontrolled NHBDs are important potential contributors to an improvement in the severe and growing organ shortage. A number of current and potential problems and concerns could limit fully developing the NHBD resource. The public also perceives similar issues and potential for problems in the NHBD donation process, as indicated by public surveys in Tallahassee, Detroit, and Philadelphia that report a lesser willingness to donate as a controlled NHBD of 22%, or as an uncontrolled NHBD of 29.2%, among those recording a willingness to donate as a heart-beating (brain-dead) donor (R.M. Arnold, personal communication, July 30, 1997). By and large, the data show that the organ procurement organizations surveyed by the IOM are doing a dedicated and increasingly successful job, along with transplant centers, in working to improve donor procurement and the state of transplantation. Nevertheless, there are some inconsistencies in the implementation of procurement programs across the nation, and improvements should be made. Given the contributions of the End Stage Renal Disease Program and other sources of federal support, the national data and organ allocation systems, the oversight and OPO standard setting of the Department of Health and Human Services, and most particularly the requirements of the U.S. Organ Procurement and Transplantation Network for national as well as local public appreciation and support of transplantation and donation, it is clear that transplantation is in many ways a nationwide effort. Recommendations to promote a more consistent and publicly explainable approach are likely, if they are appropriate and are thoughtfully implemented, to contribute to a more effective effort. This report understands the need for improvement and some national uniformity with the desirability of local initiative and responsiveness to local practice and conditions. Not all the issues that could have been explored have been addressed. Many have been left for, and deserve, future discussion. A process for involvement of the national transplant community, donor families, recipients, and the public to continue to develop policy may be desirable. In any case, given the current state of affairs and the strong desirability of, at a minimum, a coherent and defensible national approach, steps should be taken to provide some uniform national policies and improved consistency. This report provides information, analysis, conclusions, and recommendations to the sponsor, the Department of Health and Human Services, regarding the issues that the department raised as particular concerns and regarding additional issues that were identified as currently salient.

References

Alexander JW, Bennett LE, Breen TJ. Effect of Donor Age on Outcome of Kidney Transplantation. *Transplantation* 57(6):871–876, 1994.

Alvarez-Rodriguez J, del Barrio-Yesa R, Torrente-Sierra J, et al. Posttransplant Long-Term Outcome of Kidneys Obtained from Asystolic Donors Maintained Under Extracorporeal Cardiopulmonary Bypass. *Transplant Proc* 27(5):2903–2905, 1995.

Anaise D, Rapaport FT. Use of Non-Heart-Beating Cadaver Donors in Clinical Organ Transplantation—Logistics, Ethics, and Legal Considerations. *Transplant Proc* 25(2):2153–2155, 1993.

Andrews PA, Denton MD, Compton F, et al. Outcome of Transplantation of Non-Heart-Beating Donor Kidneys. *Lancet* 346:53, 1995.

Arnold RM. *Procuring Organs for Transplant: The Debate Over Non-Heart-Beating Cadaver Protocols*. Baltimore: Johns Hopkins University Press, 1995.

Arnold RM. Testimony at Public Workshop on the Medical and Ethical Issues of Maintaining the Viability of Organs for Transplantation. Washington, DC, July 30, 1997.

Arnold RM, Youngner SJ. The Dead Donor Rule: Should We Stretch It, Bend It or Abandon It? *Kennedy Institute of Ethics Journal* 3(2):263–278, 1993.

Banks GJ. Legal and Ethical Safeguards: Protection of Society's Most Vulnerable Participants in a Commercialized Organ Transplantation System. *Am J Law Med* 21(1):45–110, 1995.

Bart KJ, Macon EJ, Humphries AL, et al. Increasing the Supply of Cadaveric Kidneys for Transplantation. *Transplantation* 31(5):383–387, 1981.

Beasley CL, Capossela CL, Brigham LE, et al. The Impact of a Comprehensive Hospital-Focused Intervention to Increase Organ Donation. *J Transplant Coordination* 7(1):6–13, 1997.

Bos MA. Legal Issues Concerning the Use of Non-Heart-Beating Donors. *Transplant Proc* 27(5):2929–2932, 1995.

Braslow J. Testimony at Public Workshop on the Medical and Ethical Issues of Maintaining the Viability of Organs for Transplantation. Washington, DC, July 30, 1997.

Briceno J, Lopez-Cillero P, Ruflan S, et al. Impact of Marginal Quality Donors on the Outcome of Liver Transplantation. *Transplant Proc* 29:477–480, 1997.

Caplan AL. Requests, Gifts, and Obligations: The Ethics of Organ Procurement. *Transplant Proc* 18 (3, Suppl. 2):49–56, 1986.

Caplan AL. The Telltale Heart: Public Policy and the Utilization of Non-Heart-Beating Donors. *Kennedy Institute of Ethics Journal* 3(2):251–262, 1993.

Casavilla A, Ramirez C, Shapiro R, et al. Experience with Liver and Kidney Allografts from Non-Heart-Beating Donors. *Transplant Proc* 27(5):2898, 1995(a).

Casavilla A, Ramirez C, Shapiro R, et al. Liver and Kidney Transplantation from Non-Heart Beating Donors: The Pittsburgh Experience. *Transplant Proc* 27(1):710–712, 1995(b).

Casavilla A, Mazariegos G, Fung JJ. Cadaveric Liver Donors: What Are the Limits? *Transplant Proc* 28(1):21–23, 1996.

Chapman JR, Hibberd AB, McCosker C, et al. Obtaining Consent for Organ Donation in Nine NSW Metropolitan Hospitals. *Anaesth Intensive Care* 23(1):81–87, 1995.

Childress JF. Non-Heart-Beating Donors of Organs: Are the Distinctions Between Direct and Indirect Effects and Between Killing and Letting Die Relevant and Helpful. *Kennedy Institute of Ethics Journal* 3(2):203–216, 1993.

Cho YW, Terasaki PI, Gjertson DW, et al. A Major Source of Kidneys for Transplantation: Non-Heart-Beating Donors (unpublished). Submitted to the *N Engl J Med*, April 15, 1997.

Coolican M. Testimony at Public Workshop on the Medical and Ethical Issues of Maintaining the Viability of Organs for Transplantation. Washington, DC, July 30, 1997.

Corlett S. Public Attitudes Toward Human Organ Donation. *Transplant Proc* 7(6, Suppl. 3):103–110, 1985.

Cosio FG, Pelletier RP, Falkenhain ME, et al. Impact of Acute Rejection and Early Allograft Function on Renal Allograft Survival. *Transplantation* 63(11):1611–1615, 1997.

REFERENCES

Council on Scientific Affairs and Council on Ethical and Judicial Affairs of the American Medical Association. Persistent Vegetative State and the Decision to Withdraw or Withhold Life Support. *JAMA* 263(3):426–430, 1990.

D'Alessandro AM. Testimony at Public Workshop on the Medical and Ethical Issues of Maintaining the Viability of Organs for Transplantation. Washington, DC, July 30, 1997.

D'Alessandro AM, Hoffman RM, Knechtle SJ, et al. Controlled Non-Heart-Beating Donors: A Potential Source of Extrarenal Organs. *Transplant Proc* 27(1):707–709, 1995(a).

D'Alessandro AM, Hoffman RM, Knechtle SJ, et al. Successful Extrarenal Transplantation from Non-Heart-Beating Donors. *Transplantation* 59(7): 977–982, 1995(b).

Daemen JHC, de Wit RJ, Bronkhorst MWGA, et al. Non-Heart-Beating Donor Program Contributes 40% of Kidneys for Transplantation. *Transplant Proc* 28(1):105–106, 1996.

Daemen JHC, Oomen APA, Janssen MA, et al. Glutathione *s*-Transferase as Predictor of Functional Outcome in Transplantation of Machine-Preserved Non-Heart-Beating Donor Kidneys. *Transplantation* 63(1):89–93, 1997.

DeVita MA. Organ Donation from Non-Heart-Beating Cadavers, 1994. Pp. 33–37 in Arnold RM, et al. *Procuring Organs for Transplant: The Debate Over Non-Heart-Beating Cadaver Protocols.* Baltimore, MD: Johns Hopkins University Press, 1995.

DeVita MA, Snyder JV. Development of the University of Pittsburgh Medical Center Policy for the Care of Terminally Ill Patients Who May Become Organ Donors After Death Following the Removal of Life Support. *Kennedy Institute of Ethics Journal* 3(2):131–143, 1993.

DeVita MA, Snyder JV, Grenvikm A. History of Organ Donation by Patients with Cardiac Disease. *Kennedy Institute of Ethics Journal* 3(2):113–129, 1993.

Douglass GE, Daly M. Donor Families' Experience of Organ Donation. *Anaesth Intensive Care* 23:96–98, 1995.

Emanuel EJ. A Review of the Ethical and Legal Aspects of Terminating Medical Care. *Am J Med* 84(2):291–301, 1988.

Evans RW, Orians CE, Ascher NL. The Potential Supply of Organ Donors: An Assessment of the Efficiency of Organ Procurement Efforts in the United States. *JAMA* 267(2):239–245, 1992.

Federle MP. Milestones and Future Trends in Solid Organ Transplantation. *Radiologic Clinics in North America* 33(3):417–434, 1995.

Field DR, Gates EA, Creasy RK, et al. Maternal Brain Death During Pregnancy. *JAMA* 260(6):816–822, 1988.

Frader J. Non-Heart-Beating Organ Donation: Personal and Institutional Conflicts of Interest. *Kennedy Institute of Ethics Journal* 3(2):189–198, 1993.

Franz HG, DeJong W, Wolfe SM, et al. Explaining Brain Death: A Critical Feature of the Donation Process. *J Transplant Coordination* 7:14–21, 1997.

Gallup Organization, Inc. *The American Public's Attitudes Toward Organ Donation and Transplantation: A Survey.* Boston: The Partnership for Organ Donation, 1993.

Gortmaker SL, Beasley CL, Brigham LE, et al. Organ Donor Potential and Performance: Size and Nature of the Organ Donor Shortfall. *Crit Care Med* 24(3):432–439, 1996.

Gould L, Reddy CVR, Becker W, et al. Hemodynamic Consequences of Afterload Reduction in Patients with Valvular Abnormalities. *J Chron Dis* 33:445–458, 1980.

Grossman MD, Reily PM, McMahon D, et al. Who Pays for Failed Organ Procurement and What Is the Cost of Altruism? *Transplantation* 62(12): 1828–1831, 1996.

Halevy A, Brody B. Brain Death: Reconciling Definitions, Criteria, and Tests. *Ann Intern Med* 119(6):519–525, 1993.

Hauptman PJ, O'Connor KJ. Procurement and Allocation of Solid Organs for Transplantation. *N Engl J Med* 336(6):422–431, 1997.

Health Care Financing Administration (HCFA). "HCFA Statistics 1996—Utilization." *HCFA, the Medicare and Medicaid Agency.* On-line. Available: http://www.hcfa.gov, July 1, 1997.

Hibbard AD, Pearson IY, McCosker CJ, et al. Potential for Cadaveric Organ Retrieval in New South Wales. *British Medical Journal* 304:1339–1343, 1992.

Hoshinaga K, Fulita T, Naide Y, et al. Early Prognosis of 263 Renal Allografts Harvested from Non-Heart-Beating Cadavers Using an In Situ Cooling Technique. *Transplant Proc* 27(1):703–706, 1995.

Hoshino T, Maley WR, Bulkley GB, et al. Ablation of Free Radical-Mediated Reperfusion Injury for the Salvage of Kidneys Taken from Non-Heartbeating Donors. *Transplantation* 45(2): 284–289, 1988.

Jacobbi LM, McBride V, Etheredge EE, et al. Costs Associated with Expanding Donor Criteria: A Collaborative Statewide Prospective Study. *Transplant Proc* 29(1550–1556), 1997.

Kennedy Institute of Ethics Journal [entire] 3(2), 1993.

Kootstra G. The Asystolic, or Non-Heartbeating, Donor. *Transplantation* 63(7): 917–921, 1997.

Kootstra G. Statement on Non-Heart-Beating Donor Programs. *Transplant Proc* 27(5):2965, 1995.

Kootstra G, Daemen JHC. Procurement of Organs for Transplantation from Non-Heart-Beating Cadaver Donors in Europe. Pp. 39–53 in Arnold RM, et al. *Procuring Organs for Transplant: The Debate Over Non-Heart-Beating Cadaver Protocols.* Baltimore, MD: Johns Hopkins University Press, 1995.

Light JA, Kowalski AE, Ritchie WO, et al. Developing a Rapid Organ Recovery Program: An Innovative Solution to the Organ Donation Crisis. *UNOS Update* 10(1):5–10, 1994.

Light JA, Kowalski AE, Ritchie WO, et al. New Profile of Cadaveric Donors: What Are the Kidney Donor Limits? *Transplant Proc* 28(1):17–20, 1996.

Lynn J. Are the Patients Who Become Organ Donors under the Pittsburgh Protocol for "Non-Heart-Beating Donors" Really Dead? *Kennedy Inst Ethics J* 3(2):167–178, 1993.

Martin CC. The Uniform Anatomical Gift Act. *Am J Psychiat* 126(9):1252–1255, 1970.

Martin DK, Meslin E. The Give and Take of Organ Procurement. *J Med Philos* 19:61–78, 1994.

McMahan J. The Metaphysics of Death. *Bioethics* 9(2):91–126, 1995.

Mejia RE, Pollack MM. Variability in Brain Death Determination Practices in Children. *JAMA* 274(7):550–553, 1995.

Miller HC, Alexander JW, Smith EJ, et al. Salutary Effects of Phentolamine (Regitine) on Renal Vasoconstriction in Donor Kidneys: Experimental and Clinical Studies. *Transplantation* 17:201–210, 1974.

Miranda B. In presentation of: Beasley C, Wight C, Cohen B, et al. Donation-Related Tasks in Four Countries. *The Organ Shortage: Meeting the Challenge. Book of Abstracts from the Fourth International Society for Organ Sharing Congress and Transplant Congresses,* Washington, DC, July 8–13, 1997.

Morris JA, Slanton J, Gibbs D. Vascular Organ Procurement in the Trauma Population. *J Trauma* 29(6):782–788, 1989.

Nathan HM. Testimony at Public Workshop on the Medical and Ethical Issues of Maintaining the Viability of Organs for Transplantation. Washington, DC, July 30, 1997.

Nathan HM, Jarrell BE, Broznik B, et al. Estimation and Characterization of the Potential Renal Organ Donor Pool in Pennsylvania. *Transplantation* 51(1):142–149, 1991.

National Kidney Foundation. *Bill of Rights for Donor Families.* New York: National Kidney Foundation, Inc., 1994.

Nicholson ML. Renal Transplantation from Non-Heart-Beating Donors. *Br J Surg* 83:147–148, 1996.

Nicholson ML, Horsburch T, Doughman TM, et al. Comparison of the Results of Renal Transplantation from Conventional and Non-Heart-Beating Cadaveric Donors. *Transplant Proc* 29:1386–1387, 1997.

Orloff MS, Reed AI, Erturk E, et al. Nonheartbeating Cadaveric Organ Donation. *Ann Surg* 220(4):578–585, 1994.

Parisi JE, Kim RC, Collins GH, et al. Brain Death with Prolonged Somatic Survival. *N Engl J Med* 306(1):14–16, 1982.

Pearson IY, Zurynski Y. A Survey of Personal and Professional Attitudes of Intensivists to Organ Donation and Transplantation. *Anaesth Intensive Care* 23(1):68–74, 1995.

Perkins KA. The Shortage of Cadaver Donor Organs for Transplantation: Can Psychology Help? *Am Psychol* 42(10):921–930, 1987.

Phillips AP, Snowden SA, Hillis AN, et al. Renal Grafts from Non-Heart-Beating Donors. *BMJ* 308:575–576, 1994.

President's Commission for the Study of Ethical Problems in Medicine and Biomedical and Behavioral Research, 1983.

Reiner M. Testimony at Public Workshop on the Medical and Ethical Issues of Maintaining the Viability of Organs for Transplantation. Washington, DC, July 30, 1997.

Report of the Ad Hoc Committee of the Harvard Medical School to Examine the Definition of Brain Death. A Definition of Irreversible Coma. *JAMA* 205: 337–340, 1968.

Riether AM, Mahler E. Organ Donation: Psychiatric, Social, and Ethical Considerations. *Psychosomatics* 36(4):336–343, 1995.

Robertson JA. Policy Issues in a Non-Heart-Beating Protocol. *Kennedy Institute of Ethics Journal* 3(2):241–250, 1993.

Sadler AM, Sadler BL, Stason EB. The Uniform Anatomical Gift Act: A Model for Reform. *JAMA* 206(11):2501–2506, 1968.

Safar P. Clinical Death Symposium. *Crit Care Med* 16:919–920, 1988.

Safar P. Resuscitation of the Ischemic Brain, in Albin MS, *Textbook of Neuroanesthesia: With Neurosurgical and Neuroscience Perspectives.* New York: McGraw-Hill, 1997.

Scheinkestel CD, Tuxen DV, Cooper DJ, et al. Medical Management of the (Potential) Organ Donor. *Anaesth Intensive Care* 23(1):51–59, 1995.

Schlumpf R, Candinas D, Largiadèr F. Definition of Cardiac Death in Regard to Organ Donation from Non-Heart-Beating Donors. *The Organ Shortage: Meeting the Challenge. Book of Abstracts from the Fourth International Society for Organ Sharing Congress and Transplant Congresses*, Washington, DC, July 8–13, 1997.

Schlumpf R, Weber M, Weinreich T, et al. Transplantation of Kidneys from Non-Heart-Beating Donors: Protocol, Cardiac Death Diagnosis, and Results. *Transplant Proc* 28(1):107–109, 1996.

Sheil AGR. Ethics in Organ Transplantation: The Major Issues. *Transplant Proc* 27(1):87–89, 1995.

Siminoff LA, Arnold RM, Caplan AL, et al. Public Policy Governing Organ and Tissue Procurement in the United States: Results from the National Organ and Tissue Procurement Study. *Ann Intern Med* 123(1):10–17, 1995.

Southard JH, Belzer FO. Organ Preservation. *Annu Rev Med* 46: 235–247, 1995.

Spielman B, Verhulst S. Non-Heart-Beating Cadaver Procurement and the Work of Ethics Committees. *Camb Q of Healthc Ethics* 6:282–287, 1997.

Starzl TE, Demetris AJ. Transplantation Milestones: Viewed with One- and Two-Way Paradigms of Tolerance. *JAMA* 273(11):876–879, 1995.

Sterneck MR, Fischer L, Nischwitz U, et al. Selection of the Living Liver Donor. *Transplantation* 60(7):667–671, 1995.

Szostek M, Danielewicz R, Lahiewska B, et al. Successful Transplantation of Kidneys Harvested from Cadaver Donors at 71 to 259 Minutes Following Cardiac Arrest. *Transplant Proc* 27(5):2901–2902, 1995.

Troppmann C, Gillingham KJ, Gruessner RWG, et al. Delayed Graft Function in the Absence of Rejection Has No Long-Term Impact. *Transplantation* 61(9):1331–1337, 1996.

United Network for Organ Sharing. Non-Heartbeating Donor Procurement Attempted. *UNOS Update* 8(2):15, 1992.

United Network for Organ Sharing. Non-Heartbeating Donation on the Rise. *UNOS Update* 10(11):3–5, 1994.

United Network for Organ Sharing. *Annual Report of the U.S. Scientific Registry for Transplant Recipients and the Organ Procurement and Transplantation Network—Transplant Data: 1988–1995*. Washington, DC: Division of Transplantation, Health Resources and Services Administration, Department of Health and Human Services, 1996.

United Network for Organ Sharing. Organ Procurement and Transplantation Network data for 1996 [unpublished], 1997.

Valero R, Sánchez J, Cabrer C, et al. Organ Procurement from Non-Heart-Beating Donors Through In Situ Perfusion or Total Body Cooling. *Transplant Proc* 27(5):2899–2900, 1995.

Varty K, Veitch PS, Morgan DT, et al. Kidney Retrieval from Asystolic Donors: A Valuable and Viable Source of Additional Organs. *Br J Surg* 81:1459–1460, 1994.

Veatch RM, Pitt JB. The Myth of Presumed Consent: Ethical Problems in New Organ Procurement Strategies. *Transplant Proc* 27(2):1888–1892, 1995.

Whiting J, Golconda M, Hayes R, et al. Economic Costs of Expanded Criteria Donors in Renal Transplantation. *The Organ Shortage: Meeting the Challenge. Book of Abstracts from the Fourth International Society for Organ Sharing Congress and Transplant Congresses*, Washington, DC, July 8–13, 1997.

Wijnen RMH, Booster MH, Stubenitsky BM, et al. Outcome of Transplantation of Non-Heart-Beating Donor Kidneys. *Lancet* 345:1067–1070, 1995.

Wing AJ, Chang RWS. Non-Heart-Beating Donors as a Source of Kidneys. *BMJ* 308:549–550, 1994.

Youngner SJ, Arnold RM, for the Working Group on Ethical, Psychosocial, and Public Policy Implications of Procuring Organs from Non-Heart-Beating Cadaver Donors. Ethical, Psychosocial, and Public Policy Implications of Procuring Organs from Non-Heart-Beating Cadaver Donors. *JAMA* 269(21):2769–2774, 1993.

Youngner SJ, Landefield CS, Coulton CJ, et al. "Brain Death" and Organ Retrieval: A Cross-Sectional Survey of Knowledge and Concepts Among Health Professionals. *JAMA* 261(15):2205–2210, 1989.

APPENDIX A

Letter to the Institute of Medicine from the Department of Health and Human Services

 DEPARTMENT OF HEALTH & HUMAN SERVICES

Office of the Secretary

The General Counsel
Washington, D.C. 20201

April 30, 1997

Kenneth Shine, M.D.
President
Institute of Medicine
National Academy of Sciences
2101 Constitution Avenue, NW
Washington, DC 20418

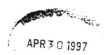

Dear Dr. Shine:

This note states the agreement between the Department of Health and Human Services and the Institute of Medicine concerning the nature and scope of IOM's inquiry regarding organ preservation and donation.

Cadaveric organ donation occurs after a determination of death under state laws. Many of these laws are modeled on the Uniform Determination of Death Act, which provides that either irreversible cessation of brain activity or irreversible cessation of respiratory and circulatory activity may be used to determine death.

With this as context, the issue under consideration is the following:

> Given a potential donor in an end-of-life situation, what are the alternative medical approaches that can be used to maximize the availability of organs from that donor without violating prevailing ethical norms regarding the rights and welfare of donors? The Institute will consider the alternative approaches, including the use of anti-coagulants or vasodilators, from the scientific as well as the ethical point of view.

It is important that the study be both timely and cost-effective. It is my understanding that you can convene advisors within two months and provide a report within four months as more fully described in the formal arrangements to follow.

For the Department, I want to thank you for your willingness to address these important issues and to lend us the benefit of your thinking.

Sincerely,

Harriet S. Rabb

APPENDIX B

Agenda and Summary of Workshop on Medical and Ethical Issues in Maintaining the Viability of Organs for Transplantation

National Academy of Sciences
Institute of Medicine
Washington, D.C.

Wednesday, July 30, 1997, Room 2004

AGENDA

Welcome and Introduction
John T. Potts, Jr., Principal Investigator

Federal Government and Political Considerations
Judith Braslow, Director, Division of Transplantation, Health Resources and Services Administration

UNOS, Procurement, Allocation, and Data Collection
Lawrence Hunsicker, President, United Network for Organ Sharing

Organ Procurement Issues in the Context of the Non-Heart-Beating Donor
Phyllis Weber, Executive Director, California Transplant Donor Network
Laurie Garretson, Executive Director, New Mexico Donor Program

Scientific Issues and Medical Perspectives
Harold Helderman, President, American Society of Transplant Physicians
Paul Terasaki, Professor of Medicine and Surgery, University of California at Los Angeles

Transplant Coordination
Mark Reiner, Past President, North American Transplant Coordinators Organization

NHBD Supply, Results, Projections, and Other Data
Howard Nathan, Executive Director, Delaware Valley Transplant Program

Consumers: Concerns of Donors and Recipients
Maggie Coolican, Volunteer Chair, National Donor Family Council
John Newmann, Past President, American Association of Kidney Patients
Lisa Kory, Executive Director, Transplant Recipients International Organization
Ron Green, heart recipient

Scientific Issues and Surgical Perspectives
Anthony D'Alessandro, University of Wisconsin Medical School

Ethical Concerns
Robert M. Arnold, Associate Professor of Medicine, University of Pittsburgh
James Childress, Professor of Religious Studies, University of Virginia Hospital

WORKSHOP SUMMARY

On July 30, 1997, the Institute of Medicine (IOM) conducted a workshop on non-heart-beating donor (NHBD) transplantation. This workshop, "The Medical and Ethical Issues in Maintaining the Viability of Organs for Transplantation" was held at the IOM and was open to the public. The principal investigator, Dr. John T. Potts, Jr., and the senior special experts were also in attendance. Dr. Potts outlined the two assumptions that formed the basis of the day's discussion. First, all possible avenues to address the inadequate donor supply should be explored and, if feasible, implemented. Second, patients that will become donors should be well cared for in an ethical manner.

Federal Government and Political Considerations

Judith Braslow of the Division of Transplantation at the Department of Health and Human Services (DHHS) highlighted the value that a group such as the senior special experts—who are not part of a transplant program but experts in their own fields of medicine, law, and ethics—can bring to a discussion of the prescribed subject matter.

Many organ procurement organizations (OPOs) are examining the potential of non-heart-beating donation programs to address the organ shortage problem. However, the ethical and medical issues involved in enhanced NHBD procurement are not clear. For this reason, the Division of Transplantation and DHHS suggested that an outside and objective party such as the IOM address these issues and assist the OPOs and transplant programs in initiating and enhancing their NHBD programs.

The important questions to be considered are the following:

- What is the state of the art of procurement and the use of NHBD organs?
- What are the ethical and medical implications of non-heart-beating donation?
- What are the timing and criteria used to make decisions about termination of life support, declaration of death, and organ preservation and recovery efforts?
- What are the rights of NHBDs?

The Division of Transplantation (DOT) is in the Health Resources and Services Administration of the DHHS. Its principal responsibilities are oversight of the Organ Procurement and Transplantation Network (OPTN) and the Scientific Registry contracts, which are both awarded to the United Network for Organ Sharing (UNOS). DOT is also responsible for efforts to increase organ donation. Towards this goal, DOT functions as a resource for the transplant community (OPOs, transplant centers, patients) and for policymakers. DOT also serves as a focal point for discussion of transplant issues. Efforts by DOT and other parts of the transplant community have resulted in increases in organ donation. From 1994 through 1996, donation increased 6.2%. However, during that same time frame, the waiting list increased by 34%. With the ever-increasing demand for organs, the transplant community has begun to use "expanded" donors, including older donors and NHBDs. Currently, NHBDs account for only 1% of the cadaver donors in a year, but it is hoped that this number can be increased. Within the DHHS there are efforts to increase organ donation through the conditions of participation of the OPOs and through managed care organizations. The Division of Transplantation has been working with several health maintenance organizations (HMOs) to inform the public about organ donation. Additionally, among the OPOs there are efforts to work both collectively and individually to improve donation.

There are many contentious issues, both medical and ethical, in the field of transplantation. Some do not apply specifically to NHBDs, for example, the allocation of organs and tissues to those on the waiting list. Others, such as the potential effect of managed care on organ transplantation, involve NHBDs more directly. Maintaining potential donors on life support can be expensive. Hospitals may be encouraged to obtain permission for removal of life support without awaiting a determination of brain death. Without an NHBD program, these potential donors are lost. Dr. Braslow presented data to support her main points. These data are included earlier in the body of this report.

UNOS: Procurement, Allocation, and Data Collection

Dr. Lawrence Hunsicker, president of UNOS, spoke about issues that affect the supply of and demand for organs. The United Network for Organ Sharing (UNOS) has a number of responsibilities:

1. Establish membership criteria for OPOs and transplant centers.
2. Develop policy for wait listing criteria and organ allocation.
3. Maintain the Scientific Registry, the data source of transplantation.
4. Increase organ donation.

With regard to organ donation, UNOS has focused on efforts to affect the "pre-donation environment." Part of that environment is the awareness of the general public about organ donation and the need for organs, and part is professional acceptance and promotion of organ donation, including understanding the needs and the role of hospital personnel in organ procurement through donor identification and maintenance. Making the general public more aware and supportive of organ donation and making families, at the appropriate time, more likely to give consent are issues that require more study, as well as better implementation in practice.

The number of cadaver organ donors is rising slightly over time, as are the number of organs procured per donor. However, these numbers do not approach the number of people currently on the waiting list or the number added yearly to the list. The number on the waiting list will expand until the number removed (through death and transplantation, or for other reasons) equals the number added. Under certain assumptions, this equilibrium might be expected at about 50,000. However, such equilibrium is not an acceptable goal since the death toll on the waiting list would be extremely high. Nor is any equilibrium likely since the character of the waiting list will change with changes in organ availability and waiting times. It can be surmised that with 50,000 people on the waiting list, the median waiting time for transplantation (the time elapsing before one-half of the people are transplanted) would be so long that many patients would never be listed.

Organ Procurement Issues in the Context of the NHBD

Phyllis Weber of the California Transplant Donor Network and Laurie Garretson of the New Mexico Donor Program discussed the day-to-day realities of procuring organs from NHBDs and the issues that OPOs face in initiating NHBD programs. One of the obstacles can be the lack of enthusiasm of their related hospitals for an NHBD program, although some hospitals would like to have such a program. Still another complication is the level of detail a hospital will tolerate in protocols from the OPOs. Some hospitals want to develop internally many or all aspects of their practice. OPOs must take these factors into consideration.

There is consistency among OPOs in some provisions of NHBD practice, but there are essentially no standards in some areas, such as where in the hospital removal from life support and cannulation procedures take place, what medications are given to donors and when they are administered, and when cannulation is performed. These areas of inconsistency put public trust at risk, but any standards developed should allow flexibility provided this does not compromise public support for NHBD programs. Protocols should be locally adopted with consultation of numerous committees including ethics and the clergy. Organizations, at this point, are often hesitant to begin programs for fear of being accused of causing or speeding the death of donors.

The crucial thing that both OPO and hospital staff need to understand is that the role of the family, and the role of staff in assisting the family, do not end with consent. The benefit to members of the family in being able to donate and provide something positive from their tragedy can be helpful in their grieving process. Because NHBD organ recovery is often more complicated, which has led to greater caution about this complexity on the part of OPO staff, it is likely that NHBD families are better informed about the procurement process than families of brain-dead donors. NHBD procedures require detailed explanations, but Ms. Weber reported that families are often ahead of the health care profession in accepting donation and the issues and complexities that are involved. OPOs involve the families in many of the decisions and share information to prevent distrust. Also, they rely on the attending physician to pronounce death and perhaps could expand this role to avoid ethical conflicts and blurring of the line between the organ donor and the dying patient. However, there has not been an attempt to come together to establish one policy, and the OPOs and their programs could benefit from some feedback on standards or guidelines for many of these issues. Both Ms. Weber and Ms. Garretson responded positively to a question about the value of recommendations for some consistent NHBD protocol provisions.

Scientific Issues and Medical Perspectives

As was mentioned by Judith Braslow of DOT, the organ shortage has brought about the use of donors accepted under expanded criteria. There have been numerous studies of the effect of these donor organs on outcomes. One of the concerns expressed by OPOs and others was the potential for reduced viability of NHBD organs. Dr. Harold Helderman, president of the American Society of Transplant Physicians (ASTP), presented workshop attendees with the results of numerous studies of the comparability of organs, particularly kidneys from NHBDs to organs from heart-beating cadaver donors. Because of the use of expanded criteria for donors, both heart-beating donor and NHBD kidneys currently tend to come from older donors, although NHBDs tend to be the older. The use of NHBDs is widespread (25 of 66 OPOs in 1994) but infrequent, accounting for only 1% of cadaver donors. These organs also tend to be from older donors and always have longer warm ischemic times than those from brain-dead donors. However, many of the data show that in the case of controlled NHBDs, this does not seem to affect graft and recipient survival rates negatively compared to heart-beating donors. Uncontrolled NHBDs are associated with a considerably higher rate of delayed graft function, but ultimately, survival of these grafts is not substantially worse than heart-beating donor graft survival.

A goal of the ASTP is the analysis and dissemination of scientific data on transplantation to inform policymaking. The ASTP put together a position statement on NHBD, with its suggestions, reservations, and goals for NHBD programs. This statement has five parts:

1. The ASTP supports and applauds all clinically and scientifically sound means of expanding the donor pool, within ethical and legal considerations.

2. The ASTP continues to subscribe wholly to the "dead donor rule" and feels that NHBDs meet those criteria.

3. The ASTP subscribes to the altruistic view of donation and to preservation of the autonomy of the donor family and wishes of the patient, if known.

4. The ASTP is opposed to the utilization of NHBDs without established protocols and procedures for retrieval that have been approved by the necessary bodies.

5. Uncontrolled NHBDs do not meet the principles of the ASTP, particularly in the area of consent, and therefore, the ASTP does not support the widespread use of this organ source. If institutions choose to pursue this donor group, they should do so under the protocols and approval of their institutional review boards.

Accompanying Dr. Helderman was Dr. Paul Terasaki of the University of California at Los Angeles. Dr. Terasaki and his colleagues have been developing a formula for meeting the growing national demand for organs. They have developed a projection of the numbers of donors from different categories that would be needed and achievable to meet the growing shortage. They suggest that in the next 10 years, if demand continues to grow at the same rate it has for the past 10 years, there will be close to 70,000 people on the waiting list for a kidney transplant. This model proposes an accelerated effort over the next four years to increase donors from all sources, including living donors, expanded donors, and NHBDs. Dr. Terasaki's data show that the risk of using older donors would be mitigated by matching them to older recipients. For the NHBD part of the effort, the model calls for 700 more NHBDs per year, nationally. After the initial four years at this level of accelerated, aggressive recruitment of donors, the model would allow for the tapering off of living donors and extended donors, with the new levels of NHBDs and heart-beating donors eventually entirely meeting the needs of patients with organ failure.

This model works on the assumption that the waiting list maintains the same rate of growth, although it is expected that as organs became more readily available, the number of waiting list members would likewise increase. However, Dr. Terasaki noted that the model's time frame could be extended or slightly upgraded to meet this potential change in the rate of growth of the waiting list. Another important contribution to this model would be passage of legislation that allows the cannulation and perfusion of donors prior to the consent of families, since kidneys from victims of trauma (emergency room deaths) have better survival rates than kidneys from NHBDs that die non-trauma-related deaths. Whatever the issues, the NHBD will play an essential role in future efforts to meet the demand for organs, according to Dr. Terasaki.

Transplant Coordination

Mark Reiner, past president of the North American Transplant Coordinators Organization (NATCO), spoke about some of the issues and concerns that have arisen in transplant coordinator work with NHBDs. Although NATCO believes that there is misinformation about NHBDs generated by the media, this has created a good opportunity for discussion. There are too many inconsistencies in the procedures for NHBDs and a need for some consensus, he believes.

The rights of the potential donor and rights of donor families to make end-of-life decisions should be no different than for any dying patient. There should be a good flow of information, and communication with the family should be supportive as well. Ideally, NATCO believes that explaining the donation process and obtaining consent for donation should be done by the transplant coordinator, accompanied by the attending physician or other hospital staff who have rapport with the family.

Other issues and concerns requiring national attention include timing and types of medications administered to NHBDs. Further study of the efficacy and effect of these drugs will be essential to decide these issues. Also, the determination of death can be a very difficult issue and is rife with conflicts of interest. The criteria to ascertain brain death are fairly well established, but prior to the reexamination of the NHBD as a source of organs, the determination of cardiac death did not require great precision. Therefore, few if any scientific studies are available, and only anecdotal information and experience remain to inform this debate. A concern was expressed that since it is less costly to end life support early, an NHBD program would encourage a decrease in the pronouncement of brain death and the procurement of the full range of organs in good condition from heart-beating donors. Managed care and other cost-containment considerations could influence this trend. The potential for a diminished supply of hearts and other extrarenal organs should be considered in the development of protocols.

NATCO supports increased use of NHBDs, but because of the issues that still must be resolved it urges careful preparation of hospital staff.

NHBD Supply, Results, Projections, and Other Information

Dr. Howard Nathan discussed his work in attempting to define the number of potential NHBDs in the United States and his efforts with the Coalition for Donation. The number of cadaver donors has increased over the past 4 years by about 12–13%. However, the number is currently at a plateau of about 1% growth per year. Dr. Nathan and his colleagues have done several reviews of medical records in different states to determine what the number of potential donors, including NHBDs, would be if all potential donors were referred to OPOs. They predict no more than 14,000 brain-dead donors and about 25,000–26,000 NHBDs, which shows the overwhelming potential of NHBDs to increase the donor pool. Even with the usual 50% consent rate, the potential is for approximately 14,000 NHBDs nationally in a given year.

These projections point up the need for some consensus on increasing the number of NHBDs. However, there are difficulties in creating and implementing nationwide policy and protocols related to the extreme diversity among OPOs. Most OPOs are separate entities from transplant programs, but 9 of the 63 OPOs are still attached to transplant programs and are actually in the hospitals. There are 15 OPOs that cover populations of more than 5 million people. The rest cover considerably fewer people. The number of hospitals that an OPO is connected with ranges from 8 to 182, and the OPOs serve from 1 to 18 transplant centers each.

According to DHHS regulations, OPOs must maintain a certain level of donor recruitment to continue to participate in Medicare and the OPTN. This level is based on the statistic of donors per million population (dmp). Many feel that this number does not account for enough of the local characteristics—cultural, social, and ethnic—of the OPOs' service areas. However, it is currently used to identify OPOs with particularly successful donor programs. These programs have been studied to determine if some of their practices could be applied nationwide for better national procurement. Such studies have not been focused on NHBDs.

An increase in NHBDs is not the only source of increasing donations in general. Dr. Nathan spoke of some local efforts in the state legislatures to boost donation. One example is the Pennsylvania law that requires hospitals to report all deaths to their OPOs at or near the time of death. This means that donors are being referred even when they may not meet brain death criteria, which had been the previous practice of OPO referrals. This routine referral law includes a fine for hospitals failing to report deaths to the OPO and has resulted in a significant increase in donors, many of them NHBDs. Illinois passed the "live and learn" legislation in 1993 that dedicated $2 million annually to public education on donor issues. Advertisements and donor card registry drives boost donor sign-up and donation. Other efforts, such as voluntary routine referral, have been successful in other areas throughout the country. These types of efforts could expand donation and solve some of the concerns about the loss of potential NHBDs who are not referred. This can happen only if OPOs have active NHBD programs. The focus of UNOS's efforts to increase public awareness of donor need is the Coalition on Donation. Dr. Nathan is the president of this organization, which was started only a few years ago. The Coalition on Donation is discussed briefly in the body of this report.

Consumer Concerns of Donors and Recipients

Ms. Maggie Coolican, from the National Donors Family Council and the mother of a young donor, spoke about the discoveries that have come from the interaction of donor families. Donor families frequently express common concerns and convictions about organ donation. The way a family is treated during the dying process of a loved one and the request for organ donation has a tremendous impact on the consent rate, as well as on its feelings about the donation afterwards. Most families express a positive feeling and benefit from the ability to give a gift during their time of tragedy, but some also feel that there is a lack of information and consideration from medical and OPO staff. Trust and belief in the medical community are essential to the continuance of an altruistic model of organ donation. Families need to be offered the opportunity to be involved in considering options and understanding what is going to happen during the procurement process.

Because families, once they have decided to donate organs, often want to have as many usable organs as possible, interventions such as catheterization and medication, when there are assurances that they will not be unduly harmful to the potential donor, are usually acceptable to the family. However, Ms. Coolican again stressed the importance of involving and informing the family about such matters.

There is evidence of many inconsistencies throughout the health care system in the practices of organ procurement and donation requests. These variations can have an effect on the trust of donor families in the care they and their loved ones received. This is an important consideration because donor families can be a strong voice in promoting organ donation. It is important that any national consensus for NHBDs be developed with collaborative efforts that involve input from the public as well as experts. Issues that should be included are consent for medication and other invasive procedures; education of the family and health professionals about the process and the reasons for particular interventions; consistency in supporting the rights of families; and making the experience of non-heart-beating donation as similar as possible to the dying process with non-donors.

Lisa Kory of the Transplant Recipients International Organization and John Newmann of the American Association of Kidney Patients spoke about the importance of public education in maintaining public trust. Public education efforts should, in general, focus on the crucial need for organs, so that when the time of decision comes, there is a base of understanding as well as a predisposition to consent. Professional education about the care of potential donors and the legal and ethical issues involved is crucial as well. Some standardization in the form of medical practice guidelines about donor care and the declaration of death could prove essential for avoiding conflicts of interest and improving public trust.

The final speaker for the donor and recipient panel was Ron Green, recipient of a heart transplant, who spoke in part for Ms. Kory. He voiced the concerns of the patient waiting for a transplant. These patients want to be assured that the organs they received are obtained under the highest ethical standards. This assurance is also important to prevent public mistrust from decreasing the consent rate and the donor pool. Standardization of OPO protocols, particularly for NHBDs, where mistrust is high following critical media reports, should be adopted in the near future. The public needs to understand that the donor's physician, and not a member of the organ recovery team, makes the decisions about critical care, and ultimately determines death. It should be generally understood that the decision to withdraw life support is made completely by the families and is separate from the potential donation. All of these issues, if standardized and well explained, will help increase public trust in non-heart-beating organ donation and organ donation in general.

Scientific Issues and Surgical Perspectives

The University of Wisconsin, where Dr. Anthony D'Alessandro is part of the organ transplant program, has a unique perspective on the NHBD issue, since it has been engaged in NHBD procurement continually since 1974. The university has averaged approximately 10% NHBDs annually since 1988.

Dr. D'Alessandro briefly outlined the procedure for NHBD organ retrieval. After the decision to terminate life support, and the second decision to donate organs, the patient is moved to the operating room (OR) for the withdrawal of life support or may remain in the intensive care unit depending on the wishes of the family to be in attendance. Cannulas are placed in the femoral arteries for the purpose of perfusion of cooling and preserving solution following the declaration of death. Prior to the removal of support, heparin (10,000–30,000 U) and phentolamine (10–20 mg) are administered. The reason for using phentolamine is to prevent vasospasm during the dying process. The program has not noted any more than minimal and transient reactions with either of these drugs, and its reading of the literature indicates no reason for expecting an adverse affect in most donors. Both drugs are utilized in other settings in higher doses than used in organ procurement. In fact, phentolamine has many positive cardiac effects. Dr. D'Alessandro believes that these drugs do not harm the patient or hasten their death.

Dr. D'Alessandro's noted that short intervals of warm ischemia do not have much impact on the long-term function of the graft. This is true in kidneys, and Dr. D'Alessandro expressed a growing comfort with moderate ischemia for livers as well. For kidneys, the initial rate of dialysis for recipients is higher in NHBD transplants than in heart-beating transplants, but the follow-up shows little or no long-term impact. In a 10-year follow-up, graft survival was 42% in NHBDs and 50% in heart-beating donors which is not a statistically significant difference. Many are skeptical about the viability of organs other than kidneys exposed to even short periods of warm ischemia. Based on his experience, Dr. D'Alessandro encouraged exploration of the potential of extrarenal organs from NHBDs. The University of Wisconsin has had success with the transplantation of livers and pancreases and has done one lung transplant from a NHBD. Dr. D'Alessandro also encourages the development of broad guidelines for NHBDs, but warns against strict national protocols that can stifle innovation. The guidelines should be beneficial to transplant centers and OPOs exploring a NHBD program, but not so burdensome as to prevent the development of these programs.

Ethical Concerns

Dr. Robert Arnold, chair of the committee that developed the Pittsburgh protocol for NHBDs in 1992, discussed three topics with major ethical ramifications in the development of any standards or guidelines for non-heart-beating donation. Because of their important ethical implications, these provisions and any others about which there are concerns should be developed and discussed with public trust as a leading objective. Dr. Arnold stressed that this meant not just gaining public trust, but really deserving it by thoroughly examining all of the areas of possible conflict of interest or appearance of impropriety.

NHBDs are currently only a small percentage of cadaver donors, but due to ongoing changes in medical practice, this percentage could increase quickly. For example, the withdrawal of life support is often happening within the first 24 to 48 hours after the critical event and before the patient can meet brain death criteria. These patients, however, are potential NHBDs, which makes a national consensus even more critical.

Determination of Death

The issue that makes procedures for the determination of death so critical in organ donation is that this determination has to be moved as close as possible in time to the cessation of cardiac function. In doing this, transplant personnel risk taking organs from patients who are not yet dead. In the Pittsburgh protocol, the standard is 2 minutes without cardiac function, and this defines the cessation as "irreversible." There are few, if any, empirical data that indicate when autoresuscitation of cardiac function is no longer possible. Dr. Arnold noted that the 2-minute definition assumes that even if the cessation could be reversed, it can be defined as irreversible because a decision has been made not to resuscitate. It is important to remember that these patients have decided, or their families have decided, that they will forgo life-sustaining treatment.

Interventions to Promote Organ Viability

Although the priority goal is to optimize the care of the dying patient, interventions are undertaken in the dying patient in most OPO protocols to promote the viability of organs. These include the use of femoral catheters, administration of medications, arterial monitoring to reliably determine death, and even the fact that death usually takes place in the OR so that procurement can begin immediately. Are there ethical barriers to these interventions if they are not for the benefit of, or might even be harmful to, the dying patient?

Conflicts of Interest

NHBD protocols and procedures have quite a bit of variation, which offers the advantage of promoting innovation but also has disadvantages. Some of the NHBD concerns truly require national standards, such as the interval of asystole that indicates irreversible loss of cardiac function. Many local hospitals do not have the medical and ethical expertise to develop and review a NHBD policy. This is worrisome because with adverse public reporting, local policies can have national impact. Consensus on the national level, involving experts in all fields of medicine applicable to this process, and public input would be particularly helpful for areas in which hospitals are most likely to face accusations of conflict of interest.

Dr. James Childress followed with some final points on applicable ethical principles for the NHBD situation. First, he drew a line between the donor patient and the donation. In most cases, the patient who is dying does not consent to organ donation. Usually the family is the donor, and the dead patient is the donation. Another consideration is the difference between the patient and the donor. Too often these terms are intermixed, and a patient often is referred to as a donor even before consent has been obtained. Dr. Childress suggested, at minimum, use of the terms donor and potential donor to distinguish between the two.

Regarding many of the issues, but particularly the concerns of treating the patient versus treating the organs, Dr. Childress encouraged the IOM to see this not as finding a balance, but as aiming for a goal within certain limitations. The goal in this case is organ procurement that can be realized within ethically acceptable limits. This reflects better the direction of the discussion of the pressing need for organs and suits better the accepted assumption that increasing organ donation is a worthy and ethical objective.

There are two ethical approaches that Dr. Childress suggested for consideration and application. First, there are other situations in medicine that might compare to organ procurement and NHBDs in terms of what can be done to a dead body and what is meant by patient benefit. These accepted values and norms might inform discussion and public understanding of non-heart-beating donation in ways that could apply to the development of standards.

Another means of looking at these issues and their ethical impact is the principle of double effect. Dr. Childress gave an example to explain this concept. In any case of care at the end of life there are accepted procedures for relieving pain and suffering, even at the risk of hastening death. The legitimate goal is relieving pain by doing what is necessary. The risk of hastening death is acceptable under the principle of double effect because it is not intended and is counterbalanced by the good effect of relieving pain. Dr. Arnold noted that this principle could be extended to viewing the preservation of donor organs as the family's good objective and accepting certain measures that further this objective even if they may pose the unintended risk of hastening death. Could this be publicly or medically accepted? What interventions would cross the line of acceptability? What cannot be done even with family consent? These questions may be answerable only with public input and both medical and ethical expertise in a process of consensus policy development. Dr. Childress did not propose accepting all his suggestions but rather including them as part of the discussion of the important issues.

Conclusion

At the end of the workshop, Dr. Potts, the principal investigator, thanked the participants and observed that their contributions had provided a most helpful and thought-provoking foundation for the analysis, findings, and recommendations of this report.

APPENDIX C

U.S. Organ Procurement Organizations and Letter of Request for Non-Heart-Beating Donor Protocols

---

See the map in Figure C.1 for the service area of each organ procurement organization.

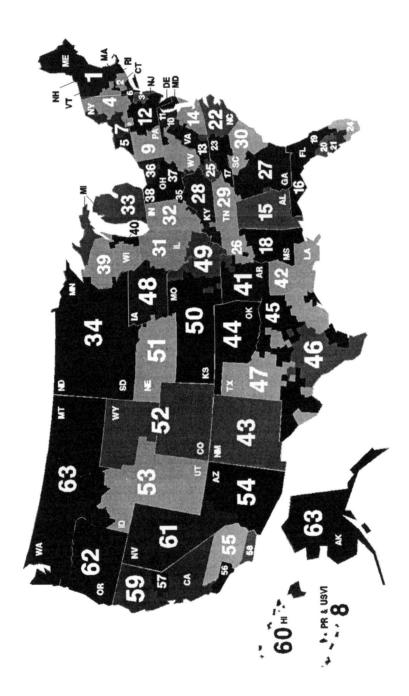

FIGURE C-1 Service areas of U.S. organ procurement organizations, 1997. SOURCE: Coralyn Colladay, Esq., Department of Health and Human Services.

1. New England Organ Bank (Newton, Mass.)
2. NorthEast Organ Procurement Organization and Tissue Bank (Hartford, Conn.)
3. New Jersey Organ and Tissue Sharing Network (Springfield)
4. Center for Donation and Transplantation (Albany, N.Y.)
5. Upstate New York Transplant Services, Inc. (Buffalo)
6. New York Organ Donor Network (New York City)
7. University of Rochester Organ Procurement Program
8. LifeLink of Puerto Rico
9. Center for Organ Recovery and Education (Pittsburgh)
10. Washington Regional Transplant Consortium (Washington, D.C.)
11. Transplant Resource Center of Maryland, Inc. (Baltimore, Md.)
12. Delaware Valley Transplantation Program (Philadelphia)
13. Virginia Organ Procurement Agency (Medlothian)
14. LifeNet (Virginia Beach, Va.)
15. Alabama Organ Center (Birmingham)
16. The Organ Procurement Organization at the University of Florida Medical Center (Gainesville)
17. LifeShare of the Carolinas (Charlotte, N.C.)
18. Mississippi Organ Recovery Agency (Jackson)
19. TransLife (Orlando, Fl.a)
20. LifeLink of Florida (Tampa)
21. LifeLink of Southwest Florida (Tampa)
22. Carolina Organ Procurement Agency (Greensville, N.C.)
23. Carolina LifeCare (Winston-Salem, N.C.)
24. University of Miami Organ Procurement Organization
25. Life Resources Regional Donor Center (Johnson City, Tenn.)
26. Mid-South Transplant Foundation, Inc. (Memphis, Tenn.)
27. LifeLink of Georgia (Atlanta)
28. Kentucky Organ Donor Affiliates (Louisville)
29. Tennessee Donor Services (Nashville)
30. South Carolina Organ Procurement Agency (Charleston)
31. Regional Organ Bank of Illinois (Chicago)
32. Indiana Organ Procurement Organization, Inc. (Indianapolis)
33. Organ Procurement Agency of Michigan (Ann Arbor)
34. Upper Midwest Organ Procurement Organization, Inc. (St. Paul, Minn.)
35. Ohio Valley Life Center (Cincinnati)
36. LifeBanc (Cleveland, Ohio)
37. Lifeline of Ohio Organ Procurement Agency, Inc. (Columbus)
38. Life Connection of Ohio (Dayton)
39. University of Wisconsin Organ Procurement Organization (Madison)
40. Wisconsin Donor Network (Milwaukee)
41. Arkansas Regional Organ Recovery Agency (Little Rock)
42. Louisiana Organ Procurement Agency (Metairie)
43. New Mexico Donor Services (Albuquerque)
44. Oklahoma Organ Sharing Network (Oklahoma City)
45. Southwest Organ Bank, Inc./Southwest Transplant Alliance (Dallas)
46. South Texas Organ Bank, Inc. (San Antonio)
47. LifeGift Organ Donation Center (Houston)
48. Iowa Statewide Organ Procurement Organization (Iowa City)
49. Mid-America Transplant Association (St. Louis, Mo.)
50. Midwest Organ Bank (Westwood, Kan.)
51. Nebraska Organ Retrieval System, Inc. (Omaha)
52. Colorado Organ Recovery Systems, Inc. (Denver)
53. Intermountain Organ Recovery System (Salt Lake City)
54. Donor Network of Arizona (Phoenix)
55. Southern California Organ Procurement Center (Los Angeles)
56. Regional Organ Procurement Agency of Southern California (Los Angeles)
57. Golden State Donor Services (Sacramento, Calif.)
58. Organ and Tissue Acquisition Center of Southern California (San Diego)
59. California Transplant Donor Network (San Francisco)
60. Organ Donor Center of Hawaii (Honolulu)
61. Nevada Donor Network, Inc. (Las Vegas)
62. Pacific Northwest Transplant Bank (Portland, Ore.)
63. LifeCenter Northwest (Seattle)

INSTITUTE OF MEDICINE
National Academy of Sciences
2101 Constitution Avenue, NW, Washington, DC 20418

Roger Herdman, M.D.,
Senior Scholar

Telephone: 202-334-1302
Facsimile: 202-334-3862
INTERNET: RHERDMAN@NAS.EDU

May 27, 1997

Dear Sir,

Very recently Secretary Shalala asked the Institute of Medicine (IOM), "given a potential donor in an end-of-life situation," to explore "what are the alternative medical approaches...including the use of anti-coagulants and vasodilators...that can be used to maximize the availability of organs from that donor without violating prevailing ethical norms regarding the rights and welfare of donors?" At issue are approaches to recovering solid organs, primarily kidneys and livers from non-heart-beating donors (NHBD).

In responding promptly to the Secretary's request, an understanding of present NHBD practices would be most helpful. The Division of Transplantation, HRSA, has kindly provided addresses of all Organ Procurement Organizations and all institutions, including yours, that have appeared on a list provided by UNOS, "Non-heart-beating Donors Recovered in the U.S. 1992-1996 By Donor Hospital." **We would greatly appreciate your sending a copy of your Non-Heart-Beating Donor Protocol(s) to me at the above address.**

The IOM is a private, scientific organization, not part of government. We will not be looking into, or reporting on, the practices of any specific institution, and we will treat your information as privileged, confidential and not to be shared with any agency. We are primarily interested in identifying the range of practices current in the United States. We will send responders copies of our report, which will be published by the National Academy Press this fall. I hope that you can provide this valuable information to help us make the best scientific and ethical study possible.

Sincerely,

Roger C. Herdman, MD